ANESTHESIA FOR THE NEW MILLENNIUM

DEVELOPMENTS IN
CRITICAL CARE MEDICINE AND ANESTHESIOLOGY

Volume 34

The titles published in this series are listed at the end of this volume.

ANESTHESIA FOR THE NEW MILLENNIUM

Modern Anesthetic Clinical Pharmacology

edited by

THEODORE H. STANLEY
AND TALMAGE D. EGAN

*Department of Anesthesiology,
The University of Utah Medical School,
Salt Lake City, Utah, U.S.A.*

SPRINGER-SCIENCE+BUSINESS MEDIA, B.V.

A C.I.P. Catalogue record for this book is available from the Library of Congress.

ISBN 978-94-010-5935-0   ISBN 978-94-011-4566-4 (eBook)
DOI 10.1007/978-94-011-4566-4

Printed on acid-free paper

TABLE OF CONTENTS

vii

Preface

Talmage D. Egan, M.D.

This volume is a summary of the proceedings of a postgraduate course in clinical anesthesiology held at Snowbird, Utah on February 19-23, 1999. Sponsored by the University of Utah School of Medicine Department of Anesthesiology and the Office of Continuing Medical Education, this course is offered annually (each year with a different focus) and is now in its 44th year. Entitled *Anesthesia for the New Millennium*, the 1999 meeting was intended to be a comprehensive review of the clinical pharmacology of anesthesia as the year 2000 approaches.

Anesthesia for the New Millennium: Modern Anesthesia Clinical Pharmacology contains the refresher course lectures of the 1999 meeting and is a review of the current state of the art in anesthesia clinical pharmacology. The authors of the individual chapters are among the world's most widely recognized experts in the pharmacology of perioperative medicine. The book features sections on new pharmacology concepts, new drug delivery techniques, recently released drugs and novel thinking about older drugs. It also addresses several areas that have recently emerged as very hot clinical and research topics including depth of anesthesia monitoring technology and anesthesia drug interactions.

This textbook's purpose is to serve as a concise, up-to-date review of the current thinking in the world of anesthesia pharmacology. Although each chapter stands by itself, collectively the chapters constitute a detailed and contemporary survey of the field. The book's quality authorship, broad scope and up-to-the-minute currency make it an excellent addition to any anesthesiologist's pharmacology reference library. As the seventeenth addition to a continuing series, I hope that this textbook will

T. H. Stanley and T. D. Egan (eds.), Anesthesia for the New Millennium, ix–x.
© 1999 *Kluwer Academic Publishers.*

help practitioners apply the recent advances in anesthesia pharmacology to the safety and well being of their patients.

The editors want to acknowledge the expert assistance of Dr. John Miner in editing the manuscripts, and of Ms. Patricia Earl in preparing them.

LIST OF CONTRIBUTORS

Peter L. Bailey, MD
Department of Anesthesiology, University of Utah Health Sciences Center, Salt Lake City, Utah, U.S.A.

Talmage D. Egan, MD
Department of Anesthesiology, University of Utah Health Sciences Center, Salt Lake City, Utah, U.S.A.

Edmond I Eger II, MD
Department of Anesthesia, University of California, San Francisco, San Francisco, California, U.S.A.

Dennis M. Fisher, MD
Departments of Anesthesia and Pediatrics, University of California, San Francisco, San Francisco, California, U.S.A.

Pierre Fiset, MD
Department of Anaesthesia, McGill University, Royal Victoria Hospital, Montreal, Quebec, Canada

Peter S.A. Glass, MB, ChB, FFA(SA)
Department of Anesthesiology, Duke University Medical Center, Durham, North Carolina, U.S.A.

Steven E. Kern, PhD
Department of Anesthesiology, University of Utah Health Sciences Center, Salt Lake City, Utah, U.S.A.

xii

Igor Kissin, MD, PhD
Department of Anesthesia, Harvard Medical School, Brigham and
Women's Hospital, Boston, Massachusetts, U.S.A.

Mervyn Maze, MB, ChB, FRCP
Department of Anesthesia, Stanford University School of Medicine, Palo
Alto Veterans Administration Medical Center, Palo Alto, California,
U.S.A.

Carl Rosow, MD
Department of Anesthesia, Harvard Medical School, Massachusetts
General Hospital, Boston, Massachusetts, U.S.A.

Peter S. Sebel, MBBS, PhD, MBA
Department of Anesthesiology, Emory University School of Medicine,
Atlanta, Georgia, U.S.A.

Theodore H. Stanley, MD
Department of Anesthesiology, University of Utah Health Sciences Center,
Salt Lake City, Utah, U.S.A.

Donald R. Stanski, MD
Department of Anesthesia, Stanford University School of Medicine,
Stanford, California, U.S.A.

Paul F. White, PhD, MD
Department of Anesthesiology and Pain Management, The University of
Texas Southwestern Medical Center, Dallas, Texas, U.S.A.

NEW PHARMACOKINETIC CONCEPTS

Peter S.A. Glass

Much of this review course is directed towards reviewing of 'New Concepts in Pharmacokinetics and Pharmacodynamics' and their application for the New Millennium. Thus this review will simply highlight some of these issues which will be discussed in greater detail in subsequent chapters. Most of the pharmacokinetic (and pharmacodynamic) principles that guide the administration of intravenous and volatile anesthetics are very similar. I will concentrate on the development of newer principles for intravenous anesthetics, but many of these are equally applicable to the volatile anesthetics.

For anesthetic drugs to be effective, they must reach their site of action within the central nervous system. In 1628 William Harvey proved in Exercitatio Anatomica De Motu Cordis Et Sanguinis In Animalibus that venous blood was transported to the arterial circulation and thus to the organs of the body by the heart. It was recognized almost immediately that this meant drugs given into veins could be rapidly carried to the entire body. Indeed, in 1657 Christopher Wren injected opium intravenously by means of a quill and bladder in dogs and man, rendering them unconscious, but Wren probably did not realize that they were "anesthetized." The practice of intravenous anesthesia has depended upon a steady improvement in the understanding of how an intravenous drug is disposed in the body (i.e. its pharmacokinetics), how these drugs affect the body (pharmacodynamics), the development of more pharmacokinetically adept drugs (i.e., designed for rapid onset and offset) and on improving technology for their administration. The culmination of these efforts has been the ability to provide closed-loop automated infusion of an intravenous drug(s) to maintain an adequate state of

1

T. H. Stanley and T. D. Egan (eds.), Anesthesia for the New Millennium, 1–11.
© *1999 Kluwer Academic Publishers.*

anesthesia (1-4). What are the concepts that have enabled these developments? I will divide them into three subgroups:

1) Application of multi-compartment pharmacokinetic models to derive dosing schemes, their application into automated drug delivery devices, and enhancement in understanding drug offset and deriving and testing of pharmacokinetic models.

2) The biophase and its inclusion in dosing schemes, defining the concentration-effect relationship and the early fingerprinting of new intravenous drugs.

3) Drug interactions, their role in the components of anesthesia and the development of monitors of these components.

MULTI-COMPARTMENT MODELS

Although multi-compartment pharmacokinetic models had been well described it was only in 1968 that Kruger-Thiemer described for the first time the infusion regimen theoretically required to quickly achieve and maintain a constant plasma concentration of an intravenously administered drug whose kinetics are described by a 2-compartment model (5). The infusion scheme described by Kruger-Theimer to maintain a target concentration was termed the **BET** scheme by Scwilden and colleagues (6). The **B** is the loading <u>b</u>olus (C_TV_1), an infusion at a rate of (C_TCl_S) to replace drug <u>E</u>liminated from the body, and an exponential decreasing infusion at a rate:

$$C_TV_1(k_{12}e^{-k_{21}t}+k_{13}e^{-k_{31}t})$$

to replace drug <u>T</u>ransferred to the peripheral tissues where C_T is the target concentration, V_1 is the volume of distribution of the central compartment, Cl_S is terminal clearance and the k's are the inter-compartmental clearances. More than a decade after publication of Kruger-Thiemer's classic paper, Schwilden and colleagues in Bonn interfaced a microcomputer to an infusion pump and demonstrated clinical application of the BET infusion scheme (7-9). Many other groups have since implemented either the BET algorithm, or modifications of this algorithm, on microcomputers connected to infusion pumps (10). These algorithms are based on polyexponential equations or compartment models and calculate the infusion rates theoretically required to obtain the desired plasma drug concentration.

Although there are minor differences in the approach taken by different investigators using pharmacokinetic model-driven infusion systems, all are conceptually similar. Each consists of a microcomputer interfaced to an infusion pump. The microcomputer executes a program that incorporates the pharmacokinetic model. In using the device, the anesthesiologist enters a target plasma or effect-site drug concentration. This target concentration is based on knowledge of the pharmacokinetic-dynamic relationship of the drug and the desired effect, as well as the individual responses of the patient. At frequent intervals (e.g., every 9-15 seconds), the program compares the target concentration with the current prediction of the plasma or effect-site drug concentration, which is computed by real-time simulation of a pharmacokinetic model of the drug being infused. The computer calculates the infusion rate required to achieve the desired target concentration and transmits this rate to the pump, after adjusting the rate to reflect the physical capabilities of the pump. The pump then delivers drug to the patient at the desired rate. As a result of the increasing popularity of intravenous anesthesia and continuous infusion techniques, the inherent reasonableness of pharmacokinetically-based drug delivery, and the promising results achieved with automated administration of a variety of drugs by research groups around the world, pharmacokinetic model-driven infusion has now become a commercial device for the administration of propofol. This system consists of a commercial pump and the "Diprifusor" software that provides the control algorithm. This device is presently available in Europe (11) and is awaiting approval in several countries including the U.S. It is expected that further devices consisting of standard infusion pumps, most of which already contain powerful microprocessors, will be equipped with the capability to perform pharmacokinetic model-driven infusions as a software-selectable option. Pharmacokinetic parameters for various drugs will be programmed into the device. The user will use the pump's keypad or soft keys to select the drug to be infused and to enter pharmacokinetically relevant information about the patient, such as weight, age, and sex, and will ensure that the infusion setup is primed with drug at a specified concentration. Then, the keypad will be used to enter target concentrations in the same manner that the dial on a calibrated vaporizer is utilized in the titration of an inhalation anesthetic. Alternatively, the pharmacokinetic model may be built into a future generation of anesthesia workstations. These workstations could then control many different brands of infusion pumps, and could provide a common platform for implementing precise titration of intravenous anesthetics in the concentration domain.

The application of pharmacokinetic parameters to determine dosing schemes led to the need to evaluate and improve the accuracy of the pharmacokinetic parameters used within automated intravenous drug delivery systems (12-17). With the goal of improving pharmacokinetic model-driven infusion device performance, Shafer et al. (16) were the first to recalculate the optimal pharmacokinetic parameters of fentanyl directly from the observed concentrations that were obtained during fentanyl administration via a pharmacokinetic model-driven infusion device, using the initial pharmacokinetics of McLean and Hug (18). He and other investigators have adapted and refined tools (such as NONMEM) that are used to derive pharmacokinetic parameters. In addition mathematical techniques such as Bayesian forecasting have been incorporated into optimizing pharmacokinetic parameters and determining population-based pharmacokinetic parameters (19). This refinement in determining pharmacokinetic parameters, combined with their practical application, has also led to a greater understanding of how dependent the derived pharmacokinetic parameters are on the mode and duration of administration. With this has come a greater understanding of the effects of age, gender, disease, cardiac bypass, etc., on drug disposition, thereby facilitating dosing regimes for these population groups (20-22).

With the application of mathematical modeling of pharmacokinetics parameters came the ability to provide simulations of the relationship between dose and drug concentration. These simulations provided an understanding of the complex interaction of elimination and redistribution and the impact of drug dose and duration on the decline in drug concentration after the termination of drug administration (23,24). The term 'Context sensitive half-time' was coined by Hughes and colleagues to describe a 50% decline in drug concentration following an infusion. They showed through simulations that the time required for a

50% decline in drug concentration was context sensitive to the duration for which the drug had been administered. As anesthesiologists are not necessarily interested in only a 50% decline, this concept has been termed the 'Context sensitive decrement time.' This concept gave practitioners a far better understanding of the factors determining offset of drug concentration and, with an understanding of drug interactions (see below), allowed a more rational means for the choice and titration of drugs intra-operatively to facilitate recovery (25). This concept combined with population-based pharmacokinetic parameters also explained differences in offset of drug effect between populations to be explained (26) (e.g., the differences in pharmacokinetic parameters for fentanyl in children leads to their having a much shorter context sensitive half-time compared to adults).

Thus the work by Kruger-Theimer in providing the mathematical description of the relationship between pharmacokinetic parameters and dosing led to several new concepts in pharmacokinetics. These included automated drug delivery, enhanced pharmacokinetic modeling for deriving pharmacokinetic parameters, and the ability to perform simulations that have led to such concepts as 'Context sensitive decrement-times'.

THE BIOPHASE

Much of the work in pharmacokinetics was directed towards plasma drug concentration and largely ignored the fact that the effect of the drug was in a site distal to the circulation, i.e. the biophase or effect compartment. Sheiner and colleagues in the early 70s began to model the relationship between drug concentration and effect (27). From this an effect compartment was proposed as part of the classical multi-compartment model. Pharmacokinetic-dynamic modeling allowed the rate constant for drug transfer between the central compartment and biophase to be determined, and from this dosing schemes could be derived to obtain target biophase concentration (and thus the desired effect). Targeting a desired effect could also be incorporated into automated drug delivery systems (28,29). Simulations of drug dose and biophase concentration demonstrated the differences in onset of drug effect between intravenous compounds (23). This has been extremely important to clinicians as this has enhanced their understanding of both dose and timing of drug administration to achieve a desired effect.

With an understanding of the biophase it has been possible and desirable to define for anesthetic drugs their concentration effect relationship (30-34). Like the concept of MAC (minimal alveolar concentration that will prevent a purposeful movement in 50% of patients to skin incision) a similar term Cp50 has been coined for intravenous anesthetics. Cp50 represents the concentration at which 50% of patients do or do not respond to a defined stimulus, e.g. respond to a verbal command. The Cp50 for the end points of analgesia, loss of consciousness, movement at skin incision during anesthesia, and suppression of the electro-encephalogram has been defined for several intravenous anesthetics.

With an enhanced understanding of pharmacokinetic modeling and the biophase, it is possible early on in drug development to predict a drug's profile. A typical example of this was in the development of remifentanil. In the initial phase 1 and 2 studies of this compound its pharmacological action as a mu opioid agonist was established. When these initial studies were performed rich pharmaco-kinetic (multiple blood samples) and pharmacodynamic assessments (analgesia/EEG) were obtained. This allowed pharmacokinetic/dynamic modeling to be performed (20,35-37). From this the likely dosing scheme for intra- and post-operative analgesia could be determined. In addition this early work brought the realization that the advantage of remifentanil would be its ability to provide high-dose intra-operative analgesia without impacting on recovery. Also the impact of age and gender on dosing of the drug was established. This early fingerprinting of a drug's pharmacokinetic/dynamic relationship allows early assessment of the drug's ultimate clinical potential and enables much more goal-directed phase 3 and 4 studies. The use of pharmacokinetic/dynamic modeling has also led to greater understanding of how changes in volumes, clearances and ke0's will affect the clinical properties of a drug in terms of onset, dosing and offset of effect. This has enhanced our understanding of our present drugs and will hopefully facilitate the development of newer compounds.

DRUG INTERACTIONS

Once the concentration-response relationship could be defined for intravenous anesthetics it was a natural progression to ascertain the impact of the interaction between opiates and hypnotics on loss of consciousness and movement at skin incision. These studies have helped in our understanding of the contributions of consciousness and analgesia in the process of anesthesia. Opioids produce only a moderate reduction in the CP50 for loss of consciousness but provide a marked reduction in the Cp50 for skin incision with propofol or the MAC of volatile anesthetics (38-40). There is a ceiling effect of the opioid in reducing the Cp50/MAC and this occurs at propofol or volatile anesthetic concentration equal to their Cp50/MAC awake value (38-45). These data indicate that anesthesia is the process of rendering a patient unconscious and then providing sufficient analgesia to inhibit noxious stimuli from reaching the brain and causing a return towards consciousness (see chapter on drug interactions for a more complete discussion). This concept has led to the idea that to monitor the state of anesthesia it may be necessary to separate hypnosis from analgesia. The Bispectral monitor was being developed at the same time as these concepts were evolving. It thus became apparent that a monitor of brain activity was more likely to provide information on sedation and consciousness than analgesia. Studies have now confirmed that the Bispectral index provides a good predictor of consciousness and can be used to facilitate titration of anesthetics to enhance intra-operative care and recovery (46-48).

The past 20 years have resulted in numerous new concepts in pharmacokinetics and pharmacodynamics. These have had a very practical impact on the delivery of anesthesia from the development of Target Controlled Intravenous anesthesia delivery systems to more rational drug choices and enhanced drug dosing.

REFERENCES

1. Schwilden H, Stoekel H, Schuttler J: Closed-loop feedback control of propofol anaesthesia by quantitative EEG analysis in humans. Br J Anaesth 62: 290-296, 1989

8

2. Schwilden H, Schüttler J, Stoekel H: Closed-loop feedback control of methohexital anesthesia by quantitative EEG analysis in humans. Anesthesiology 67: 341, 1987

3. Struys M, Smet T, Audenaert S, Versichelen L, Mortier E, Rolly G: Development of a closed loop system for propofol using bispectral analysis and a patient-individual pharmacokinetic-dynamic (PK-PD) model. Preliminary results. Brit J of Anaesthesia 78 Suppl 1: 23, Abs A.76, 1997

4. Kenny GNC, Davies FW, Mantzardis H, Fisher AC: Closed-loop control of anesthesia. Anesthesiology 77((3)): A328, 1992

5. Kruger-Thiemer E: Continuous intravenous infusion and multicompartment accumulation. Eur J Pharmacol 4: 317-324, 1968

6. Schwilden H: A general method for calculating the dosage scheme in linear pharmacokinetics. Eur J Clin Pharmacol 20: 379-386, 1981

7. Schwilden H, Schuttler J, Stoekel H: Pharmacokinetics as applied to total intravenous anaesthesia: theoretical considerations. Anaesthesia 38((suppl)): 51-52, 1983

8. Schwilden H, Stoekel H, Schuttler J, Lauven PM: Pharmacological models and their use in clinical anaesthesia. Eur J Anaesth 3: 175-208, 1986

9. Schüttler J, Schwilden H, Stoekel H: Pharmacokinetics as applied to total intravenous anaesthesia: practical implications. Anaesthesia 38((suppl)): 53-56, 1983

10. Glass PSA, Shafer SL, Jacobs JR, Reves JG: Intravenous drug delivery systems, Anesthesia. Edited by Miller R. New York, NY, Churchill Livingstone, 1994, pp 389-416

11. Servin FS: TCI compared with manually controlled infusion of propofol: a multi-center study. Anaesthesia 53(Supplement 1): 82-6, 1998

12. Raemer DB, Buschman A, Johnson MD: Alfentanil pharmacokinetic model applied to ambulatory surgical patients: does a computerized infusion improve predictability? Anesthesiology 69: A243, 1988

13. Raemer DB, Buschman A, Varve JR: The prospective use of population pharmacokinetics in a computer-driven infusion system for alfentanil. Anesthesiology 73: 66, 1990

14. Glass PSA, Goodman DK, Ginsberg B, Reves JG, Jacobs JR: Accuracy of pharmacokinetic model-driven infusion of propofol. Anesthesiology 71(3A): A277, 1989

15. Coetzee JF, Glen JB, Wium CA, Boshoff L: Pharmacokinetic model selection for target controlled infusions of propofol. Assessment of three parameter sets. Anesthesiology 82(6): 1328-45, 1995

16. Shafer SL, Varvel JR, Aziz N, Scott JC: The pharmacokinetics of fentanyl administered by computer controlled infusion pump. Anesthesiology 73: 1091-1102, 1990

17. Ausems ME, Stanski DR, Hug CC: An evaluation of the accuracy of pharmacokinetic data for the computer assisted infusion of alfentanil. Br J Anaesth 57: 1217-1225, 1985
18. McClain DA, Hug CC, Jr.: Intravenous fentanyl kinetics. Clin Pharmacol Ther 28: 106, 1980
19. Maitre PE, Stanski DR: Bayesian forecasting improves the prediction of intraoperative plasma concentrations of alfentanil. Anesthesiology 69: 652-659, 1988
20. Minto CF, Schnider TW, Egan TD, et al.: The influence of age and gender on the pharmacokinetics and pharmacodynamics of remifentanil. I. Model development. Anesthesiology , 1997
21. Bailey JM, Mora CT, Shafer SL: Multicenter study of perioperative ischemia research group: Pharmacokinetics of propofol in adult patients undergoing coronary revascularization. Anesthesiology 81: 1288-97, 1996
22. Fiset P, Mathers L, Engstrom R, Fitzgerald D, Brand SC, Hsu F, Shafer SL: Pharmacokinetics of computer controlled alfentanil administration in children undergoing cardiac surgery. Anesthesiology 83: 944-55, 1995
23. Shafer SL, Varvel JR: Pharmacokinetics, pharmacodynamics, and rational opioid selection. Anesthesiology 74: 53-63, 1991
24. Hughes MA, Glass PSA, Jacobs JR: Context-sensitive half-time in multicompartment pharmacokinetic models for intravenous anesthetic drugs. Anesthesiology 76: 334-341, 1992
25. Vuyk J, Mertens MJ, Olofsen E, Burm AGL, Bovill JG: Propofol Anesthesia and rational opioid selection. Anesthesiology 87: 1549-62, 1997
26. Ginsberg B, Howell S, Glass PSA, Margolis JO, Ross AK, Dear GL, Shafer SL: Pharmacokinetic model-driven infusion of fentanyl in children. Anesthesiology 85: 1268-1275, 1996
27. Sheiner LB, Stanski DR, Vozeh S, Miller RD, Ham J: Simultaneous modeling of pharmacokinetics and pharmacodynamics: application to d-tubocurarine. Clin Pharm Ther 25: 358-371, 1979
28. Shafer SL, Gregg K: Algorithms to rapidly achieve and maintain stable drug concentrations at the site of drug effect with a computer controlled infusion pump. J Pharmacokinet Biopharm 20: 147-169, 1992
29. Jacobs JR, Williams EA: Algorithm to control "effect compartment" drug concentrations in pharmacokinetic model-driven drug delivery. IEEE Trans Biomed Eng 40((10)): 993-999, 1993
30. Ausems ME, Hug CC, Jr., Stanski DR, Burm AGL: Plasma concentrations of alfentanil required to supplement nitrous oxide anesthesia for general surgery. Anesthesiology 65: 362-373, 1986
31. Glass PSA, Doherty M, Jacobs JR, Goodman D, Smith LR: Plasma concentration of fentanyl, with 70% nitrous oxide, to prevent movement at skin incision. Anesthesiology 78: 842-847, 1993

32. Vuyk J, Engbers FHM, Lemmens HJM, Burm AGL, Vletter AA, Gladines MPRR, Bovill JG: Pharmacodynamics of propofol in female patients. Anesthesiology 77: 3-9, 1992

33. Scott JC, Ponganis KV, Stanski DR: EEG quantitation of narcotic effect: The comparative pharmacodynamics of fentanyl and alfentanil. Anesthesiology 62: 234-241, 1985

34. Scott JC, Cooke JE, Stanski DR: Electroencephalographic quantitation of opioid effect: comparative pharmacodynamics of fentanyl and sufentanil. Anesthesiology 74: 34, 1991

35. Egan TD, Lemmens HJM, Fiset P, Muir KT, Hermann D, Stanski DR, Shafer S: The pharmacokinetics and pharmacodynamics of GI 87084B. Anesthesiology 77(3): A369, 1992

36. Egan TD, Lemmens MH, Fiset P, Stanski DR, Shafer S: Pharmacokinetic-dynamic fingerprinting in the early development of GI87084B. Clin Pharmacol Ther 53(2): 209, 1993

37. Glass PSA, Hardman D, Kamiyama Y, Quill TJ, Marton G, Donn KH, Grosse CM, Hermann D: Preliminary pharmacokinetics and pharmacodynamics of an ultra-short-acting opioid: Remifentanil (GI87084B). Anesth & Analg 77: 1031-40, 1993

38. Vuyk J, Lim T, Engbers FHM, Burm AGL, Vletter AA, Bovill JG: The pharmacodynamic interaction of propofol and alfentanil during lower abdominal surgery in female patients. Anesthesiology 83: 8-22, 1995

39. Smith C, McEwan AI, Jhaveri R, Wilkinson M, Goodman D, Canada A, Glass PSA: Reduction of propofol Cp50 by fentanyl. Anesthesiology 77(3a): A340, 1992

40. Katoh T, Ikeda I: The effects of fentanyl on sevoflurane requirements for loss of consciousness and skin incision. Anesthesiology 88: 18-24, 1998

41. Brunner MD, Braithwaite P, Jhaveri R, McEwan AI, Goodman DK, Smith LR, Glass PSA: The MAC reduction of isoflurane by sufentanil. Br J Anaesth 72: 42-46, 1994

42. Lang E, Kapila A, et al.: The reduction of the MAC of isoflurane by remifentanil. Anesthesiology 85: 721-728, 1996

43. McEwan AI, Smith C, Dyar O, Goodman D, Glass PSA: Isoflurane MAC reduction by fentanyl. Anesthesiology 78: 864-869, 1993

44. Sebel PS, Glass PSA, Fletcher JE, Murphy MR, Gallagher C, Quill T: Reduction of the MAC of desflurane with fentanyl. Anesthesiology 76: 52-59, 1992

45. Westmoreland C, Sebel PS, Groper A, Hug CC, Jr.: Reduction of isoflurane MAC by fentanyl or alfentanil. Anesthesiology 77((3)): A394, 1992

46. Gan TJ, Glass PS, Windsor A, Payne F, Rosow C, Sebel P, Manberg P: Bispectral index monitoring allows faster emergence and improved recovery from propofol, alfentanil, and nitrous oxide anesthesia. Anesthesiology 87: 808-815, 1997

47. Glass PSA, Bloom M, Kearse L, Rosow C, Sebel P, Manberg P: Bispectral analysis measures sedation and memory effects of propofol, midazolam, isoflurane, and Alfentanil in healthy volunteers. Anesthesiology 86: 836-47, 1997
48. Lui J, Singh H, White PF: Electroencephalograph bispectral analysis predicts the depth of midazolam-induced sedation. Anesthesiology 84: 64-9, 1996

THE BIOPHASE CONCEPT

Donald R. Stanski

Lecture Objectives: To introduce clinicians to the essential role of the biophase in understanding the relationship between concentration and response, and thus the relationship between drug dose and drug response.

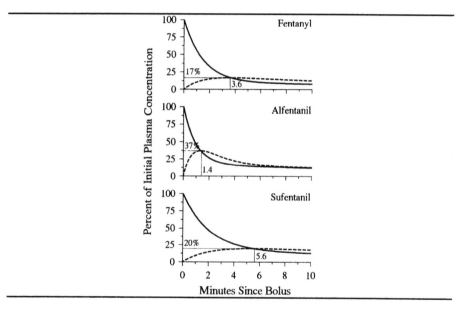

Figure 1. The plasma (solid) and biophase concentrations (dashed lines) following a bolus of 3 common opioids.

PLASMA-EFFECT SITE EQUILIBRATION

Although the plasma concentration following an intravenous bolus peaks nearly instantaneously, no anesthesiologist would induce a patient with an intravenous bolus of a hypnotic and immediately intubate the patient. The reason, of course, is that although the plasma concentration peaks almost instantly, additional time is required for the drug

13

T. H. Stanley and T. D. Egan (eds.), Anesthesia for the New Millennium, 13–18.
© *1999 Kluwer Academic Publishers.*

14

concentration in the brain to rise and induce unconsciousness, as shown in figure 1. This delay between peak plasma concentration and peak concentration in the brain is called hysteresis. Hysteresis is the clinical manifestation of the fact that the plasma is usually not the site of drug action, only the mechanism of transport. Drugs exert their biological effect at the "biophase," also called the "effect site," which is the immediate milieu where the drug acts upon the body, including membranes, receptors, and enzymes.

The concentration of drug in biophase cannot be measured. First, it is usually inaccessible, at least in human subjects. Second, even if we could take tissue samples, the drug concentration in the microscopic environment of the receptive molecules will not be the same as the concentration grossly measured in, say, ground brain or CSF. Although it is not possible to measure drug concentration in the biophase, using rapid measures of drug effect we can characterize the time course of drug effect. Knowing the time course of drug effect, we can characterize the rate of drug flow into and from the biophase. Knowing these rates, we can characterize the drug concentration in the biophase in terms of the steady-state plasma concentration that would produce the same effect. Starting with the 3 compartment model, we can now incorporate the biophase as an additional "effect compartment," as shown in figure 2.

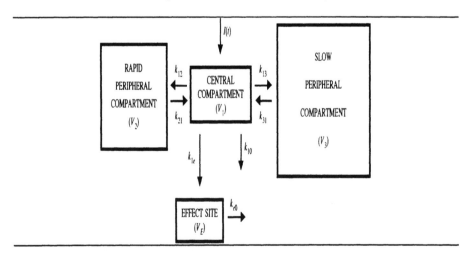

Figure 2. The compartmental model, now with an added effect site. k_{e0} is often directed outside, as though drug were eliminated from the effect site.

The effect site is the hypothetical compartment that relates the time course of plasma drug concentration to the time course of drug effect, and k_{e0} is the rate constant of drug elimination from the effect site. By definition the effect compartment receives such small amounts of drug from the central compartment that it has no influence on the plasma pharmacokinetics.

If a constant plasma concentration is maintained, then the time required for the biophase concentration to reach 50% of the plasma concentration ($t \_ k_{e0}$) can be calculated as $0.693 / k_{e0}$. Following a bolus dose, the time to peak effect site concentration is a function of *both* the plasma pharmacokinetics and k_{e0}. For drugs with a very rapid decline in plasma concentration following a bolus (e.g., adenosine, with a half-life of several seconds), the effect site concentration will peak within several seconds of the bolus, regardless of the k_{e0}. For drugs with a rapid k_{e0} and a slow decrease in concentration following bolus injection (e.g., pancuronium), the time to peak effect site concentration will be determined more by the k_{e0} than by the plasma pharmacokinetics. k_{e0} has been characterized for many drugs used in anesthesia (1-7). Equilibration between the plasma and the effect site is rapid for thiopental (9), propofol (13), and alfentanil (11); intermediate for fentanyl (11), and sufentanil (12), and the nondepolarizing muscle relaxants (1); and slow for morphine and ketorolac.

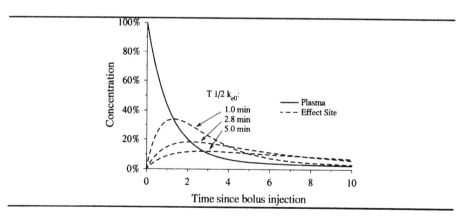

Figure 3: The plasma and effect site concentrations for propofol, assuming a $t \_ k_{e0}$ of 1, 2.8 (the real value) and 5 minutes.

Using the intravenous hypnotic propofol, we can consider the influence of k_{e0} on the onset of drug effect. Figure 3 shows the plasma concentrations and apparent biophase concentrations after an IV bolus of propofol for three values for t _ k_{e0}: 1 min, 2.8 min (the actual value for propofol) (1), and 5 min. Regardless of the value of k_{e0}, the pattern remains the same. The plasma concentration peaks (nearly) instantly and then steadily declines. The effect site concentration starts at 0 and increases over time until it equals the (descending) plasma concentration. The plasma concentration continues to fall, and after that moment of identical concentrations, the gradient between the plasma and the effect site favors drug removal from the effect site and the effect site concentrations decrease.

Examining the different values of t _ k_{e0} in figure 3 shows that as t _ k_{e0} increases, the time to reach the peak apparent biophase concentration also increases. Concurrently, the magnitude of the peak effect site concentration relative to the initial plasma concentration decreases because slower equilibration between the plasma and biophase allows more drug to be distributed to other peripheral tissues.

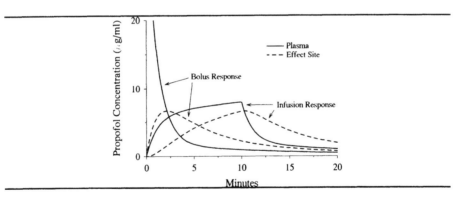

Figure 4. The plasma and effect site concentrations following a bolus or infusion of propofol.

Figure 4 shows the plasma concentrations and the apparent biophase concentrations after a bolus and 10 min infusion of propofol. The degree of disequilibrium is less after an infusion than after a bolus. Thus, during an infusion the observed drug effect parallels the plasma drug concentration to a greater extent than after a bolus.

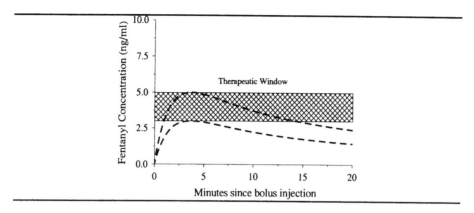

Figure 5: The effect site concentrations over time for doses of fentanyl that target the high and low edges of the therapeutic window.

Let us now integrate the sigmoidal relationship between concentration and effect, the concept of the therapeutic window, and the equilibration delay between the plasma and the site of drug effect. One must first identify, preferably with full concentration-response relationships, the edges of the therapeutic window. One can then produce dosage regimens that produce concentrations within the therapeutic window at the site of drug effect. The technique will be discussed below for intravenous drugs. One need also consider the rate of onset, as a small dose will result in a slower onset to a given effect than a larger dose. However, a larger dose will be more likely to exceed the therapeutic window, and possible cause toxic effects. For example, figure 5 shows the biophase concentrations after two different bolus doses of fentanyl designed to achieve the high and low edges of the therapeutic window for supplementing an induction with thiopental. The larger dose of fentanyl produces a rapid onset of drug effect and adequate biophase concentrations for several minutes. The biophase concentration from the lower dose momentarily brushes against the lower edge of the therapeutic window.

To conclude, the biophase is an essential concept in understanding the pharmacodynamics of the intravenous anesthetics. Clinicians intuitively understand the time course of plasma-biophase equilibration because we time our induction doses so that we intubate patients at peak biophase concentrations. As new drugs are introduced into clinical practice, understanding the plasma-effect site equilibration will lead to more rational use of these drugs

REFERENCES

1. Sheiner LB, Stanski DR, Vozeh S, Miller RD, Ham J: Simultaneous modeling of pharmacokinetics and pharmacodynamics: application to d-tubocurarine. Clin Pharmacol Ther 25:358-371, 1979

2. Hull CJ, Van Beem HB, McLeod K, Sibbald A, Watson MJ: A pharmacodynamic model for pancuronium. Br J Anaesth 50:1113-23, 1978

3. Homer TD, Stanski DR: The effect of increasing age on thiopental disposition and anesthetic requirement. Anesthesiology 62:714-24, 1985

4. Stanski DR, Maitre PO: Population pharmacokinetics and pharmacodynamics of thiopental: the effect of age revisited. Anesthesiology 72:412-22, 1990

5. Buhrer M, Maitre PO, Crevoisier C, Stanski DR: Electroencephalographic effects of benzodiazepines. II. Pharmacodynamic modeling of the electroencephalographic effects of midazolam and diazepam. Clin Pharmacol Ther 48:555-67, 1992

6. Scott JC, Stanski DR: Decreased fentanyl/alfentanil dose requirement with increasing age: a pharmacodynamic basis. J Pharmacol Exp Ther 240:159-66, 1987

7. Scott JC, Cooke JE, Stanski DR: Electroencephalographic quantitation of opioid effect: comparative pharmacodynamics of fentanyl and sufentanil. Anesthesiology 74:34-42, 1991

8. Donati F: Onset of action of relaxants. Can J Anaesth 35:S52-58, 1988

9. Dyck GB, Shafer SL: Effects of age on propofol pharmacokinetics. Seminars in Anesthesia 11:2-4, 1992

HANDEDNESS IN ANESTHETIC PHARMACOLOGY

Talmage D. Egan

The historical beginnings of stereochemistry are a fascinating piece of scientific detective work dating back to the early career of French chemist Louis Pasteur in the 1840s. Pasteur, then a young man, was interested in crystallography. While examining the crystals of tartaric acid salts with a hand lens, he serendipitously noticed that sodium ammonium tartrate existed as two distinct kinds of crystals that were mirror images of each other. After laboriously separating the right and left handed forms of the crystals into two piles, Pasteur discovered that, while the original mixture had been optically inactive, each individual pile of crystals rotated polarized light when dissolved in solution. Furthermore, the specific rotations of the two solutions were exactly equal but opposite in direction!

Based on this surprising discovery, Pasteur correctly postulated, although he could not prove, that the molecules making up the crystals were also mirror images of each other but were otherwise identical. The implication of this idea was that identical molecules with different spatial configurations might behave differently as evidenced by their effect on polarized light. From this coincidental beginning, stereochemistry has slowly emerged as an important branch of organic chemistry with profound biologic ramifications.

The mention of the word "stereochemistry" to most physicians brings back nomenclature nightmares from the lonely hours spent studying organic chemistry textbooks. Although the nomenclature

Authors Note: This chapter was adapted with permission from Egan TD: Stereochemistry and Anesthetic Pharmacology: Joining Hands With the Medicinal Chemists. Anesth Analg 1996; 83:447-50

T. H. Stanley and T. D. Egan (eds.), Anesthesia for the New Millennium, 19–29.
© *1999 Kluwer Academic Publishers.*

nuances are not particularly important, stereochemistry, and more specifically chirality, are more relevant to anesthesia practice today than ever before and are certainly more pertinent than we ever dreamed they could be when studying organic chemistry as undergraduate students.

In its broadest sense, stereochemistry is the study of how molecules are structured in three dimensions. Chirality is a unique subset of stereochemistry. Taken from the Greek word *cheir* (meaning hand), chiral is the term used to designate a molecule that has a center (or centers) of three dimensional asymmetry. The appropriateness of the term's Greek origin is clear when considering that our hands are perhaps the most common example of chirality. While they are mirror images of one another, our hands cannot be superimposed. Similarly, chirality in molecular structure results in a set of mirror image molecular twins that cannot be superimposed. This kind of molecular handedness in biologic systems is ubiquitous in nature and is almost always a function of the tetrahedral bonding characteristics of the carbon atom (1).

Chirality is thus the structural basis of enantiomerism. Enantiomers are a pair of molecules that exist in two forms that are mirror images of one another but cannot be superimposed one upon the other (1). Enantiomers are in every other respect chemically identical. Because a pair of enantiomers shares the same molecular weight, melting point, etc., they can only be distinguished *in vitro* by the direction in which, when dissolved in solution, they rotate polarized light, either dextro (d or +) or levo (l or -) rotatory (hence, the term "optical" isomers). When the two enantiomers are present in equal proportions they are collectively referred to as a racemic mixture, a mixture that does not rotate polarized light because the optical activity of each enantiomer is canceled by the other. Adding additional confusion to the molecule naming exercise, a second nomenclature system based on absolute configuration employs the designations sinister (S) and rectus (R), depending on how the molecules are sequenced (3). A partial list of important stereochemistry terms is displayed in Table 1.

Although two enantiomers cannot be easily differentiated *in vitro* except by how they rotate polarized light, when examined *in vivo* for their pharmacologic properties, two enantiomers can be distinguished in a host of ways.   This is because the molecular interactions that are the mechanistic foundation of drug action and disposition occur in three dimensions and therefore can be altered by stereochemical asymmetry (4). The schematic "lock and key" hypothesis of enzyme-substrate interplay implies that biologic systems are inherently chiral.   The pharmacologic extension of this notion is that drugs can be expected to interact with other biologic components in a geometrically specific way.   Thus, pharmacologically, not all enantiomers are created equal! Drug-cellular receptor, drug-metabolic enzyme and drug-protein binding interactions are virtually always three dimensionally exacting.   As illustrated in Figure 1, one enantiomer may be better than the other in interacting with a pharmacologic protein such as a cellular receptor or metabolic enzyme. Conceptualized in geometrical terms, one enantiomer may simply "fit" the pharmacologic protein more intimately.

TABLE 1   SOME STEREOCHEMICAL TERMINOLOGY

Stereoisomers: molecules with identical groups of atoms that are different in terms of the spatial arrangement.

Chirality: the underlying geometry of an object or molecule that allows the existence of enantiomers. The term is derived from the Greek word for hand (*Cheir*). The hands are chiral and constitute a pair of enantiomers.

Enantiomers: two molecules that bear a three-dimensional mirror image relationship to each other; also referred to as optical isomers.

Racemate: a 1:1 mixture of enantiomers.

Stereospecific: a process that makes an _absolute_ distinction between enantiomers (e.g., when one enantiomer is pharmacodynamically active and the other is not).

Stereoselective: a process that makes a *relative* distinction between enantiomers (e.g., two enantiomers that are metabolized at different rates).

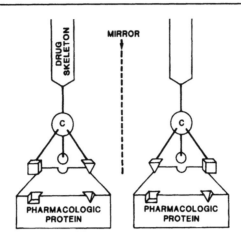

Figure 1. A schematic summarizing the implications of chirality on drug-pharmacologic protein interplay. One enantiomer of the racemic pair may be more effective than the other at binding and interacting with the pharmacologic protein (e.g., a metabolic enzyme, cellular receptor, etc.) C = chiral carbon

The implications of chirality thus span the entire pharmacokinetic-pharmacodynamic spectrum. Enantiomers can exhibit differences in absorption and bioavailability, distribution and clearance, potency and toxicology (5-9). Enantiomers can even antagonize one another across this pharmacologic spectrum (10). Adding additional complexity, enantiomers can undergo chiral inversion to the other enantiomer, and drug interactions can also be stereoselective (11-13).

When a pharmacologic process discriminates in a relative fashion between enantiomers (e.g., such as one enantiomer being metabolized more rapidly than the other), it is termed stereoselective. If the discrimination is absolute (e.g., such as one enantiomer being completely incapable of producing drug effect), the process is termed stereospecific (see Table 1).

While it is not something we think about in everyday practice, the issue of chirality applies to a surprisingly diverse array of anesthetic drugs. The sedative hypnotics thiopental, methohexital, and ketamine are administered as racemates. The inhaled agents halothane, enflurane, isoflurane and desflurane also have a center of molecular asymmetry, as do the local anesthetic agents mepivacaine, prilocaine and bupivacaine. The analgesics ibuprofen, ketorolac and methadone are also cases in point.

For some of these chiral anesthetic drugs in widespread clinical use there are important implications arising from their chirality. For example, the S(+) enantiomer of ketamine is known to be more potent than the R(-) form and is also less likely to produce psychotic emergence reactions (14-16). Figure 2 illustrates the marked pharmacokinetic and pharmaco-dynamic differences between ketamine enantiomers. Similarly, in addition to pharmacokinetic differences, the cardiac toxicity of bupivacaine is thought to be predominantly due to the d-bupivacaine enantiomer (17-19). Figure 3 illustrates the pronounced differences in the cardiac toxicity of the bupivacaine enantiomers when administered to rodents. The d-bupivacaine enantiomer produces malignant dysrhythmias and circulatory collapse at the doses studied.

In view of this enantiomeric duality, it is perhaps not surprising to discover that many of the drugs recently released into clinical anesthesia have chiral centers but have been developed as pure enantiomers. Ropivacaine, a close structural relative of bupivacaine, does not appear to have a propensity for the cardiac toxicity associated with bupivacaine, at least in part because it was developed as a single enantiomer that is theoretically less prone to be toxic to the heart (20). Cisatracurium, another example of fine tuning chirality to pharmacologic advantage, is the R-R′ optical isomer of atracurium in the *cis-cis* configuration (more nomenclature nightmares!) that does not release histamine and therefore is not associated with the cardiovascular side effects of atracurium (21).

Other drugs recently released were perhaps developed in part because their structures were non-chiral and thus the scientific complexities of chirality did not apply. Sevoflurane, for example, is the first inhaled anesthetic approved for use that has a non-chiral structure (22). Similarly, remifentanil, a new esterase metabolized opioid also exists in a single form because it does not have a center of molecular asymmetry (23).

Interestingly, nature's own anesthetic pharmacopoeia is also mindful of chirality. Perhaps without being cognizant of it, anesthetists have been administering pure enantiomeric forms of chiral drugs from

24

the earliest days of our specialty. Morphine sulfate (actually l-morphine) and d-tubocurarine are notable examples. Because these drugs are synthesized by nature's stereospecific enzymatic machinery, they exist in a single form before they are extracted and purified.

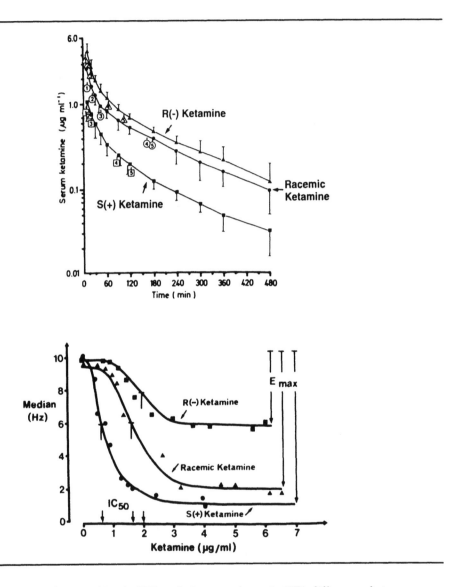

Figure 2. Pharmacokinetic (PK) and pharmacodynamic (PD) differences between ketamine enantiomers. The upper panel contrasts the concentration vs. time curves (PKs) of the enantiomers and the racemate after intravenous administration in doses sufficient to produce maximal EEG changes. The bottom panel illustrates the differences in the concentration-effect relationships (Pos) for the three "drugs."

panel illustrates the differences in the concentration-effect relationships (Pos) for the three "drugs."

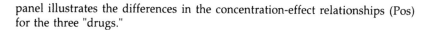

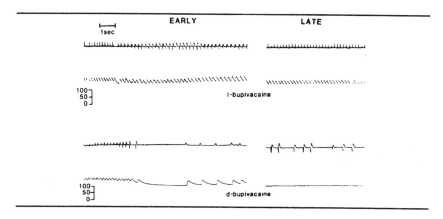

Figure 3. Representative EKG and arterial blood pressure recordings when rats received either l-bupivacaine or d-bupivacaine (2 mg/kg). The d-bupivacaine rats all experienced severe bradycardia, progressive hypotension, apnea and death. The cardiopulmonary effects in the l-bupivacaine group were less pronounced.

Undoubtedly, the emphasis on chirality in clinical pharmacology is here to stay. We have witnessed an explosion of enantiomer specific investigation in the last decade. While about a third of drugs currently in use are chiral drugs and are administered as a racemate, this percentage is likely to decline in future years (24). Pharmaceutical companies have become acutely aware of chirality's importance and are likely to shy away from the scientific ambiguities associated with the development of racemic drugs (25,26). Moreover, regulatory agencies are encouraging enantiomer specific investigation and development by more closely scrutinizing racemic compounds (27). The widespread acknowledgment of stereochemistry's importance is evident in the publication of *Chirality*, a scientific journal specially devoted to the pharmacological, biological and chemical consequences of molecular asymmetry (28).

As one might expect, the significance of stereochemistry in drug development has moved beyond the scientific laboratory, attracting the attention of Wall Street investors and the business world in an impressive fashion. There are now several pharmaceutical companies that specialize in the development of single enantiomeric forms of previously approved racemic drugs and also novel compounds. These companies have special expertise in stereochemical synthesis, separation and assay and they attract investor capital for drug development based or the public's perception of the promising future of stereochemically sophisticated drugs. The seemingly arcane and esoteric concept of chirality in drug development has become such common knowledge among educated non-medical people that it has been featured in popular magazines of the lay press (29).

Recognizing the importance of stereochemistry in clinical pharmacology today, why was chirality not as important to our practice 25 years ago? While we understood the theoretical implications of chirality at that time, the technology necessary to demonstrate the pharmacologic differences of enantiomers was not widely available. Advances by chemists in stereospecific separation and assay were required before the widely suspected theoretical importance of chirality could be confirmed (30-32). Equally important, the technology enabling the synthesis of industrial quantities of pure enantiomer was necessary to make the clinical administration of such drugs a practical reality (33,34). The ability of medicinal chemists to distinguish the subtle nuances of chiral structure in drug synthesis and assay is indeed an impressive scientific feat (35).

Having for the most part achieved these advances in stereospecific separation, assay and synthesis, the focus on the importance of chirality in pharmacology over the last decade has prompted some experts to suggest that experiments performed with racemic mixtures are of little or no value. Viewing a racemic mixture as a drug that is 50% impure, some experts have disparagingly referred to the less active or inactive enantiomer as "stereochemical ballast" (5). In what has become a widely cited and classic editorial addressing the pharmacology of chirality, Ariens suggested that experiments performed using racemic mixtures are little more than "sophisticated scientific nonsense" (36). It is quite possible to make a cogent theoretical argument that studies on racemic mixtures may be fatally flawed if the enantiomers have different pharmacodynamic activity or their concentrations decline at different rates.

Does this mean that the volumes of carefully performed scientific work describing the clinical pharmacology of anesthetics that are administered as racemic mixtures such as thiopental are clinically useless? Of course not! Lamenting the fact that some of the clinical pharmacology database upon which we base our practice was completed at a time when stereospecific synthesis and assay were not widely practical gets us nowhere, especially when these drugs continue to be administered successfully as racemic mixtures. Instead, as a specialty we now recognize that advances in stereochemistry have enabled us to refine our anesthetic pharmacology knowledge base.

We can expect to see a great deal more enantiomer specific investigation in the future. It is conceivable that such work may change the way we use some of our racemic anesthetics. At the very least we can expect that all new drugs released into clinical practice will be scrutinized for the implications of asymmetry in molecular structure.

It is astonishing that the advance of science has brought the clinical relevance of chirality in our specialty into clear focus in just a few decades. Not long ago we suspected the importance of chirality but did not have the tools to confirm it. Now, we not only know of its significance but have also begun to exploit it to our pharmacologic advantage. Having joined hands with the medicinal chemists, we have moved the pharmacology of chirality from the drawing board into the clinic. As its Greek etymology suggests, chirality is in our hands now (37).

REFERENCES

1.   Mason S: The origin of chirality in nature. Trends Pharmacol Sci 1986;7:20-23
2.   Hegstrom RA. Konderpudi DK: The handedness of the universe. Sci American 1990;262:98-105
3.   Morrison RT. Boyd RN: Organic Chemistry. 3rd Edition. Boston: Allyn and Bacon, 1973
4.   Testa B: Mechanisms of chiral recognition in xenobiotic metabolism and drug-receptor interaction. Chirality 1989;1:7-9
5.   Ariens EJ: Chirality in bioactive agents and its pitfalls. Trends Pharmacol Sci 1986;7:200-205
6.   Tucker GT, Lennard MS: Enantiomer specific pharmacokinetics. Pharmac Ther 1990;45:309-329
7.   Williams KM: Chirality: pharmacokinetics and pharmacodynamics in 3 dimensions. Clin Exp Pharmacol Physiol 1989:16:465-470
8.   Drayer DE: Pharmacodynamic and pharmacokinetic differences between drug enantiomers in humans: an overview. Clin Pharmacol Ther 1986;40:125-133

9. Lee EJD, Williams KM: Chirality. Clinical pharmacokinetic and pharmacodynamic considerations. Clin Pharmacokinet 1990;18:339-345

10. Wahlstrom G, Norberg L: A comparative investigation in the rat of the anesthetic effects of the isomers of two barbiturates. Brain Res 1984;310:261-267

11. Kaiser DG, van Geissen GJ, Reisher RJ, Wechter WJ: Isomeric inversion of ibuprofen (R)-enantiomer in humans. J Pharma Sci 1976;65:269-273

12. O'reilly RA, Trager WF, Rettie AE, Goulart DA: Interaction of amiodarone with racemic warfarin and its separated enantiomorphs in humans. Clin Pharmacol Ther 1987;42:290-294

13. Whelan E, Wood AJ, Koshakji R, Shay S, Wood M: Halothane inhibition in propranolol metabolism is stereoselective. Anesthesiology 1989;71:561-564

14. Schuttler J, Stanski DR, White PF, Trevor AJ, Horai Y, Verotta D, Sheiner LB: Pharmacodynamic modeling of the EEG effects of ketamine and its enantiomers in man. J Pharmacokin Biopharm 1987;15:241-253

15. White PF, Ham J, Way WL, Trevor AJ: Pharmacology of ketamine isomers in surgical patients. Anesthesiology 1980; 52:231-239

16. White PF, Schuttler J, Shafer A, Stanski DR, Horai Y, Trevor AJ: Comparative pharmacology of the ketamine isomers-studies in volunteers. Br J Anaesth 1985;57:197-203

17. Rutten AJ, Mather LE, McLean CF: Cardiovascular effects and regional clearances of IV bupivacaine in sheep: enantiomeric analysis. Br J Anaesth 1991;67:247-256

18. Denson DD, Behbehani MM, Gregg RV: Enantiomer-specific effects of an intravenously administered arrhythmogenic dose of bupivacaine on neurons of the nucleus tractus solitarius and the cardiovascular system in the anesthetized rat. Regional Anesth 1992;17:311-316

19. Rutten AJ, Mather LE, McLean CF, Nancarrow C: Tissue distribution of bupivacaine enantiomers in sheep. Chirality 1993;5:485-491

20. McClure JH: Ropivacaine. Br J Anaesth 1996;76:300-307

21. Lien CA, Belmont MR, Abalos A, Eppich L, Quessy S, Abou-Donia MM, Savarese JJ: The cardiovascular effects and histamine-releasing properties of 51W89 in patients receiving nitrous oxide/opioid/barbiturate anesthesia. Anesthesiology 1995;82:1131-1138

22. Smith I, Nathanson M, White PF: Sevoflurane a long awaited volatile anaesthetic. Br J Anaesth 1996;76(3):435-45

23. Egan TD: Remifentanil pharmacokinetics and pharmacodynamics: a preliminary appraisal. Clin Pharmacokinet 1995;29:80-94

24. Millership JS, Fitzpatrick A: Commonly used chiral drugs: a survey. Chirality 1993;5:573-576

25. Lennard MS: Clinical pharmacology through the looking glass: reflections on the racemate vs. enantiomer debate. Br J Clin Pharmacol 1991;31:623-625

26. Gross M, Cartwright A, Campbell B, Bolton R, Holmes K, Kirkland K, Salmonson T, Robert JL: Regulatory requirements for chiral drugs. Drug Info J 1993;27:453-457

27. Nation RL: Chirality in new drug development-clinical pharmacokinetic considerations. Clin Pharmacokinet 1994;27:249-255

28. Wainer IW, Caldwell J, Testa B: Joining hands. Chirality 1989;1:1

29. Bulls, pills and patents. The Economist. June 28, 1997 pg. 69

30. Hermansson J, Grahn A: Optimization of the separation of enantiomers of basic drugs-retention mechanisms and dynamic modification of the chiral bonding properties on an alpha 1-acid glycoprotein column. J Chromatog 1995;694:57-69

31. Soini H, Riekkola ML, Novotny MV: Chiral separations of basic drugs and quantitation of bupivacaine enantiomers in serum by capillary electrophoresis with modified cyclodextrin buffers. J Chromatog 1992;608:265-274

32. Cook CE, Seltzman TB, Tallent CR, Wooten JD III: Immunoassay of racemic drugs: a problem of enantioselective antisera and a solution. J Pharmacol Exp Ther 1982;220:568-573

33. Sheldon RA: The industrial synthesis of pure enantiomers. Drug Info J 1990;24:129-139

34. Mosher HS, Morrison JD: Current status of asymmetric synthesis. Science 1983;221:1013-1019

35. Egan TD: Stereochemistry and anesthetic pharmacology: joining hands with the medicinal chemists. [editorial] Anesth Analg 1996;83:447-450

36. Ariens EJ: Stereochemistry, a basis for sophisticated nonsense in pharmacokinetics and clinical pharmacology. Eur J Clin Pharmacol 1984;26:663-668

37. Mather LE: "Chirality is in your hands" Bull Aust NZ College of Anaesthetists 1994;3:26-32

ANESTHETICS AND VENTILATORY DRIVE

Peter L. Bailey

INTRODUCTION

Adverse respiratory effects of anesthetics are associated with some of the most serious negative outcomes in anesthesia (1). Regardless of the anesthetics or analgesic strategies employed, there is a well-documented risk for and occurrence of post-operative adverse respiratory events in 0.1-1.0% of surgical patients. Clinicians need useful information concerning respiratory drive and drug effects in order to administer medications in a rational manner and minimize the frequency with which adverse outcomes occur. This presentation will summarize current understanding of:

1) respiratory drive and rhythm generation,
2) assessing the effects of drugs on respiratory drive,
3) current knowledge concerning the effects of drugs on respiratory drive.

GENERATION OF RESPIRATORY DRIVE AND RHYTHM

Breathing is a fundamental physiologic process controlled by efferent signals from the nervous system. For clinicians, the "black box" approach to comprehending how respiratory rhythm is generated and controlled still is as useful as most other approaches. Although much work has been performed concerning the phenomenon of breathing, the molecular, synaptic, cellular and network activities that govern respiratory control in humans remain poorly described. Until single neuron activity can be measured routinely and non-invasively in humans, animal models will continue to serve as surrogates. For example, *en bloc* brainstem/

T. H. Stanley and T. D. Egan (eds.), Anesthesia for the New Millennium, 31–47.
© *1999 Kluwer Academic Publishers.*

spinal cord preparations and medullary slice models generate a respiratory rhythm in vitro and allow useful observations of the cellular and synaptic physiology of the control of breathing.

The brainstem contains several anatomically distinct groups of neurons involved in various aspects of the control of breathing, including central chemosensation, afferent signal processing, rhythm generation, and motor pattern coordination. Recent studies point to a single site, called the pre-Botzinger Complex (pBC), as containing predominantly inspiratory neurons (2). This site is critical for respiratory rhythmogenesis. Convincing evidence includes lines of investigation determining that neurons in the pBC fire before all other respiratory-related neurons and that pBC neurons drive heretofore considered rhythmogenesis centers, such as the caudal ventral respiratory group (cVRG) of neurons. Furthermore, transection studies in the rat *en bloc* in vitro preparation confirm the primary role of the pBC in respiratory rhythmogenesis.

Synaptic interactions between pBC respiratory neurons involve excitatory amino acids acting on AMPA channels whose normal function is essential for respiratory rhythmogenesis. Synaptic inhibition mediated by GABA or glycine is not essential for respiratory rhythmogenesis. The cellular basis of pBC rhythmogenesis requires an understanding of the electrophysiological, biochemical and synaptic properties of neurons within the pBC. Delineating work is currently being performed.

HOW SHOULD WE MEASURE RESPIRATORY DRIVE?

Feedback loops important to the neural regulation of minute ventilation depend on chemosensation. Oxygen tension is directly sensed in the blood at the level of the peripheral chemoreceptor. Carbon dioxide tension is indirectly sensed, via changes in pH, at numerous ventral brainstem sites. Hence, over the years, physiological, clinical and pharmacological investigations have sought to examine and define respiratory drive through techniques that permit quantification of the ventilatory responses to hypoxia *or* hypercapnia. Clinically, most often, hypoxia and hypercapnia occur simultaneously. However, the ability to interpret the significance of investigative findings is limited when neither oxygen nor carbon dioxide is held steady (clamped). Thus, the vast majority of investigations employ either hypoxic or hypercapnic methods as a means to stimulate breathing and assess respiratory drive and drug effects.

CARBON DIOXIDE AS THE PRIMARY RESPIRATORY STIMULUS

It is widely believed that the central chemosensation of CO_2 is very important to respiratory control. Physiologically, the partial pressure of CO_2 represents the primary signal in the feedback loop in respiratory homeostasis. Central chemoreceptors have widespread brainstem locations at or just rostral to the ventral medullary surface and at deeper sites near the nucleus tractus solitarius and locus caeruleus. Focal hypercapnia induces changes in pH which augment whole respiratory center output. The exact molecular nature of chemosensation remains undetermined (3).

REBREATHING VERSUS STEADY STATE METHODS

To this day, how best to quantify the ventilatory response to carbon dioxide remains controversial (4). Although such debates may seem esoteric or academic, key issues concerning the validity and significance of different methods for determining the ventilatory response to carbon dioxide and associated drug effects remain contested. For example, compared to steady state techniques, rebreathing methodologies may overestimate ventilatory drive (5). In addition, whereas steady state techniques often detect only a shift of the ventilatory response to CO_2, rebreathing techniques often detect both a shift and a depression of the slope of the ventilatory response to CO_2 (6,7). Others argue that the two methods are similar (8). Possible differences between the two methodologies may in part be related to changes in cerebral blood flow which accompany rebreathing techniques but not steady state methodologies (9).

There are numerous challenges and potential problems associated with the measurement of the ventilatory response to carbon dioxide as a primary measure of respiratory drive. These include the fact that CO_2 is quite stimulating and elicits many generalized (e.g., dyspnea, anxiety, headache) and specific (e.g., increased cerebral blood flow) reflexes or sensations. As an investigator I have frequently had the opportunity to personally experience hypercapnia in the research setting. I have always been impressed at how stressful hypercapnia (e.g., end-tidal CO_2 = 60 mm Hg) is in the drug-free state. Equally impressive is how little stress the same degree of hypercapnia induces after numerous pharmacologic treatments (see below).

Supporters and critics of both the steady state and rebreathing methods propose abundant arguments for and against each method. The rebreathing method is certainly more practical and easier to perform. Because the ventilatory response to CO_2 can be performed in 5-7 minutes, it lends itself to study design. The steady state method, which clamps CO_2 at a hypercapnic level for 15-20 minutes, has its proponents as the more valid test, but is frequently less practical, especially in the clinical research setting. Debate is likely to continue as to which test is preferable. Complicating matters is the fact that additional methodologies continue to be evaluated and employed (10). Combined with methodological differences in how investigators perform these tests, a significant lack of standardization will persist and plague our ability to interpret reports and compare results among various publications.

HYPOXIC VENTILATORY DRIVE

Although the partial pressure of oxygen does *not* significantly influence ventilatory drive under normal conditions, there has been a great deal of interest in measuring the effect of hypoxia on ventilatory drive. For clinicians this interest stems from the belief (hope?) that hypoxia, as a secondary signal in the feedback loop of respiratory homeostasis, will protect our patients from respiratory depression and serious adverse effects. Evidence supporting this is lacking.

Testing hypoxic ventilatory drive seems more risky than hypercapnic drive because of the inherent risks of hypoxia. Testing HVR is also technically challenging for several reasons, including the need to control the partial pressures of both CO_2 and O_2 during the tests. Weil (11) first developed and reported the use of progressive isocapnic hypoxia testing. Hypoxic ventilatory responses (HVR) were curvilinear and required either a hyperparabolic equation or an exponential function to describe them. For most clinicians, these mathematical representations did not easily lend themselves to clinical interpretation. The use of the method applied by Weil and colleagues presented difficulties that prevented it from becoming popular.

Rebuck and Campbell (12) developed a method which allowed a linear plot (easier to analyze than a hyperparabolic response) of the ventilatory response to hypoxia. Since both the ventilatory response to hypoxia as well as the paO_2 – SpO_2 relationship are curvilinear, plotting ventilation versus SpO_2 results in a linear plot. This allows quantification of the response by the position and slope of a line.

A most significant potential problem with these and other methodologies is that the ventilatory response to hypoxia is actually biphasic (13). The initial acute hypoxic ventilatory response (AHVR) develops and peaks within 3-5 minutes of the onset of acute hypoxia. If hypoxia persists, this peak response diminishes over the next 10 minutes (hypoxic ventilatory decline, HVD). The mechanisms underlying HVD remain to be determined and could be multifactorial. HVD mechanisms could include attenuation of carotid body chemosensation, cerebral alkalosis related to hypoxia-induced increases in cerebral blood flow, direct CNS depression by hypoxia, or changes in the concentrations and effects of central inhibitory and excitatory neurotransmitters. Methodologies that measure the HVR beyond 3-5 minutes but do not take this biphasic response into account will produce a hybrid measurement, difficult to interpret. Many studies in the past have the AHVR measured contaminated by HVD. Another confounding factor, among many, is that AHVR and HVD are altered if hypoxic challenges are repeated frequently (within day testing) without adequate time for recovery between tests. The administration of oxygen in between hypoxic challenges shortens recovery time for the HVR (14). Patients suffering from chronic hypoxia may also have their hypoxic responses attenuated (15).

WHAT DO WE KNOW (OR NEED TO KNOW) ABOUT THE EFFECTS OF DRUGS ON RESPIRATORY DRIVE?

With an understanding of the potential for anesthetics and analgesics to depress either the ventilatory response to CO_2 or hypoxia, clinicians can assess some of the risk involved when administering each drug. As in the past, 1) reports, employing various methodologies, will continue to appear in the literature, and 2) clinicians need to be able to incorporate evaluations of both new and older agents into their working body of knowledge.

Besides neuromuscular blockers (for obvious reasons) opioids represent the class of drugs which, when administered alone, are most likely to produce troublesome respiratory depression. Other intravenous agents, including sedative-hypnotics such as propofol, and anxiolytic-amnestics such as midazolam possess respiratory depressant actions which are milder and more variable than those induced by opioids (16). Importantly, combining different classes of drugs, e.g., opioids and benzodiazepines, is now recognized as perhaps the most likely approach to result in pharmacologic synergism and exaggerated effects (17). That the potent inhaled agents produce dose-dependent depression of the ventilatory response to CO_2 is well accepted. More controversial is the question "at what minimal concentration does the ability of potent inhaled anesthetics to depress the AHVR disappear?" (18-20) Because residual amounts of the older potent inhaled anesthetics could persist for a significant period of time after anesthesia, the question was of clinical interest. The use of newer less soluble potent inhaled agents should decrease any threat these anesthetics may possess to reduce the ability of patients to mount a ventilatory response to hypoxia (21). The remainder of this presentation will focus on the respiratory pharmacology of opioids.

Endogenous opioid peptides are widely distributed in brainstem nuclei regulating respiration (22). High concentrations of opiate receptors have been found in many of the supraspinal brain respiratory centers including the nucleus tractus solitarius, nucleus retroambigualis and nucleus ambiguus (23,24). Specific chemo-sensitive brain areas also mediate opioid-induced respiratory effects (22,25). Opioids interfere with pontine and medullary respiratory centers that regulate respiratory rhythmicity.

All mu-receptor stimulating opioids cause dose-dependent depression of respiration in humans (26), primarily through a direct action on brain stem respiratory centers (27,28). Controversy persists as to whether different subclasses of mu opioid receptors have disparate roles in opioid-induced respiratory depression (29). How the various respiratory centers involved with ventilatory drive, respiratory rhythm generation, chemoreception, and neural integration are affected by opioids is also unclear. The stimulatory effect of CO_2 on ventilation is significantly reduced by opioids. Thus, the slopes of the ventilatory and occlusion pressure responses to CO_2 are decreased, and minute ventilatory responses to increases in $PaCO_2$ are shifted to the right. In addition, the apneic threshold and resting end-tidal pCO_2 are increased by opioids.

Opioids also decrease hypoxic ventilatory drive (30-32). In fact, carotid body chemoreception and hypoxic drive are blunted or eliminated by low, analgesic doses of opioids. Opioids also blunt the increase in respiratory drive normally associated with increased loads such as increased airway resistance (30).

Respiratory rate is usually drastically slowed in overt opioid overdose, although hypoxic CNS insult can counter this effect. Opioids can usually be titrated to effect, especially in anesthetized patients, by observing dose-dependent decreases in the spontaneous respiratory rate. However, respiratory rate, especially in the postoperative setting, cannot serve as a reliable index of the magnitude of opioid-induced respiratory depression (23,33). High doses of opioids usually eliminate spontaneous respirations without necessarily producing unconsciousness. Patients receiving high doses of opioids may still be responsive to verbal command and often breathe when directed to do so.

Opioid-induced effects on the control of respiratory rhythm and pattern include increased respiratory pauses, delays in expiration, irregular and/or periodic breathing, and decreased, normal, or increased tidal volume. The prolonged expiratory time in the respiratory cycle induced by opioids frequently results in greater reductions in respiratory rate than tidal volume. Fentanyl depresses respiratory drive, phase timing, and activation of respiratory muscles, whereas enflurane decreases only respiratory drive (34).

Peak onset of respiratory depression after an analgesic dose of morphine is slower than after comparable doses of fentanyl, 30 ± 15 minutes versus 5 to 10 minutes (26). This is due in part to the lower lipid solubility of morphine. Because of its low lipid solubility, plasma concentrations and onset of action of morphine are nearly identical after intravenous and intramuscular administration (35). Thus, it could be argued that the selection of morphine as an IV analgesic is not the most rational choice for acute pain control in the immediate postoperative period.

Respiratory depression induced by small doses of morphine usually lasts longer than after equipotent doses of fentanyl (36). Downes et al. found that intravenous fentanyl (100 and 200 ug•70 kg^{-1}) results in a somewhat shorter period of respiratory depression than an equipotent dose of meperidine (65 to 75 mg•70 kg^{-1}) (37). These investigators also noted a faster onset and peak effect after fentanyl than meperidine (37). Even though fentanyl has a shorter onset and quicker recovery than morphine and meperidine, small doses (2 mg•kg^{-1}) produce respiratory depression for longer than is generally appreciated (more than one hour). Sufentanil (0.1 to 0.4 ug•kg^{-1}) produces shorter-lasting respiratory depression and longer-lasting analgesia than fentanyl (1.0 to 4.0 ug•kg^{-1}) (38).

Although fentanyl (4-8 ug•kg^{-1}) given during induction of anesthesia does not usually produce troublesome respiratory depression, some investigators have found significant residual respiratory depression 5 or more hours later (32,39). Recovery from the ventilatory effects of fentanyl closely parallels the decline of plasma levels (40). Large or repeated doses or continuous infusions increase the time required for lower plasma levels (below the threshold for significant respiratory effects) to be established. Plasma fentanyl concentrations of 1.5 to 3.0 ng•ml^{-1} are usually associated with significant decreases in CO_2 responsiveness (41).

Pharmacokinetic data predict and studies have demonstrated that both alfentanil and sufentanil allow more rapid recovery of respiratory function than fentanyl (42). Alfentanil has more rapid receptor dissociation kinetics than other opioids, making respiratory depression less likely after it is employed in anesthesia (43). Although adequate spontaneous ventilation after alfentanil-nitrous oxide is likely with plasma alfentanil concentrations of less than 200 ng/ml (44), significant residual respiratory depression can exist at lower levels. The effects of remifentanil, no matter what the dose, dissipate rapidly and completely within 5 to 15 minutes following termination of its administration. The pharmacodynamic effects of alfentanil, sufentanil, and remifentanil on respiratory function are not significantly different from those of fentanyl.

A review of the respiratory effects of neuraxial opioids is beyond the scope of this presentation. It is interesting to note that intrathecal morphine was introduced to clinical practice prior to adequate study of its impact on respiratory drive (33). The effects of intrathecal morphine on the ventilatory response to hypoxia in humans have just been determined in our laboratory for the first time and will be presented. (Lu, unpublished data)

FACTORS AFFECTING OPIOID INDUCED RESPIRATORY DEPRESSION

We all recognize, however, that both respiratory pharmacology and our patients are complicated and dynamic. Both drug interactions and patient conditions (normal and pathologic) can play key roles in causing troublesome respiratory depression.

Many factors can change both the magnitude and duration of respiratory depression after opioids. Patients who are sleeping are usually more sensitive to the respiratory depressant effects of opioids (45,46). Even small doses of opioids markedly potentiate the normal right shift of the $PaCO_2$-alveolar ventilation curve that occurs during natural non-rem sleep (45,46). For several days postoperatively, sleep is associated with hypoxemia (47). The mechanisms and implications of postoperative sleep disturbances are complex and relate not only to respiratory problems but also to cognitive and hemodynamic disturbances (48). Both sleep and morphine relatively spare the diaphragmatic but decrease the thoracic (rib cage) component of breathing (49). Sleep also impairs tonic and phasic upper airway muscle activity that accompanies breathing (50). This can be troublesome when patients have an opioid-based anesthetic and an operation that results in little or no postoperative pain. In such patients, apparently adequate breathing can become insufficient with the onset of asleep. In patients with conditions that impair abdominal breathing or airway function, such as those with marked obesity or sleep apnea, an increased risk of adverse respiratory events is likely with the administration of opioid analgesia.

Older patients are more sensitive to the anesthetic (51) and respiratory depressant effects of opioids (52). Older patients experience higher plasma concentrations of opioids administered on a weight basis

(35). Although older patients tend to have a lower blood volume than younger patients, the precise reason for higher plasma concentrations after similar doses is unknown. Conflicting reports argue for or against differences in pharmacokinetics (decreased clearance, increased elimination half-life) and/or pharmacodynamics (increased brain sensitivity) as the basis for the presence or absence of age-related increases in sensitivity to fentanyl (53). Older patients also have more frequent apnea, periodic breathing, and obstruction after morphine than young adults (54).

Morphine alone produces greater respiratory depression on a weight basis in neonates than adults. Its low lipid solubility normally limits blood-brain barrier (BBB) penetration. In neonates and infants with incomplete BBBs, morphine easily penetrates the brain. Neonates are not unduly sensitive to the more lipid soluble opioids (meperidine, fentanyl, sufentanil) because penetration of these drugs into the brain is not affected by BBB maturity (55). Endogenous opioid activity may also be increased in the neonate and possibly contributes to the depressed ventilatory response to hypoxia observed in such young individuals. Support for this hypothesis comes from studies demonstrating that naloxone shortens the apneic phase and stimulates the response to hypoxia in newborns but not older infants (22).

The respiratory depressant effects of opioids are increased and/or prolonged when administered with other CNS depressants, including the potent inhaled anesthetics (56), alcohol (52), barbiturates (52), benzodiazepines (38), and most of the intravenous sedatives and hypnotics. Drug interactions and synergistic depression of the ventilatory response to hypercarbia and/or hypoxia can result in bradypnea or apnea. Exceptions are droperidol, scopolamine and clonidine, which do not enhance the respiratory depressant effects of fentanyl or other opioids (37,57-60). Sedation and sleep may accompany a_2-adrenergic agonists and possibly explain some of their reported mild respiratory depressant actions (60).

Pain, particularly surgically induced pain, is thought to counteract the respiratory depressant effects of opioids. However, the contrary has been suggested by some (61,62). For example, certain post-surgical breathing patterns are not predominately determined by the level or mode of pain relief (63). Acute pain does not reverse the depression of the ventilatory response to hypoxemia which is produced by sedation with sevoflurane (64). A recent investigation of the effect of experimental pain on ventilatory control suggests that pain causes a chemoreflex-independent increase in tonic ventilatory drive (65).

It is interesting to note that while some acute tolerance to opioid-induced respiratory depression can develop, 5 to 8 months of opioid exposure may be necessary for significant tolerance to the respiratory depressant actions of opioids on hypoxic ventilatory responses to develop (22). Cross-tolerance to the respiratory depressant actions between different opioids also may be neither complete nor predictable (23). Infants of mothers on methadone maintenance demonstrate impaired central chemosensitivity to CO_2. They may also be at higher-than-normal risk for sudden infant death syndrome.

Although opioid action is usually dissipated via redistribution and hepatic metabolism rather than urinary excretion (see section on pharmacokinetics), adequacy of renal function may influence duration of opioid activity. It was previously thought that with renal insufficiency, the more potent respiratory depressant properties of the morphine metabolite M-6-glucuronide would become evident as it accumulated (66). However, a recent study indicates M-6-glucuronide is a somewhat weaker respiratory depressant than morphine (67). Nevertheless, morphine or meperidine and/or some of their metabolites can accumulate in patients with renal insufficiency and result in greater respiratory depression (see below).

Hypocapnic hyperventilation has been shown to enhance and prolong postoperative respiratory depression after fentanyl (10 and 25 mg•kg^{-1}) (32). Intraoperative hypercarbia produces the opposite effects (68). Possible explanations for these findings include increased brain opioid penetration (increased unionized fentanyl with hypocarbia) and removal (decreased cerebral blood flow with hypocarbia). Decreased liver clearance related to decreased cardiac output and hepatic blood flow may also explain this phenomenon. Also, intraoperative hyperventilation depletes carbon dioxide stores and can result in a post-hyperventilation hypoventilation syndrome. Following hyperventilation, carbon dioxide stores are repleted. This process removes CO_2 from the blood and lowers minute ventilatory requirements, resulting in hypoventilation. In this circumstance a normal $PaCO_2$ does not necessarily indicate normal or adequate minute ventilatory volumes. In patients who hyperventilate because of anxiety and/or pain, even small doses of IV opioids can result in transient apnea because of acute shifts in apneic thresholds.

Some authors suggest that the administration of opioids in anesthesia leads to increased respiratory problems (69,70). However, the vast majority of studies performed to date have failed to isolate perioperative opioid administration as particularly associated with increased respiratory problems (71). Although Beard et al. (68) found an increase in adverse respiratory events in the recovery room associated with the use of muscle relaxants and fentanyl, the frequency of a serious problem with fentanyl was rare (1/886 patients). In another study, patients receiving intravenous morphine for postoperative pain after a general anesthetic experienced more respiratory side effects than those who received regional anesthesia. Interestingly, desaturations of significance were always associated with sleep and related to obstruction, paradoxic breathing or slow respiratory rates (72). The analgesic dose of morphine used in the latter study was large (>12 mg•70 kg^{-1} IM).

CONCLUSIONS

It is convenient, but not very illuminating, to consider respiratory drive mechanisms as a "black box." Although much work has been done determining the neurophysiology and pharmacology of breathing, investigators remain limited by the models available to them. Nevertheless, valuable information can be gained from reports evaluating respiratory drive and determining the impact of anesthetics. Information learned from these reports can help clinicians develop a rational basis for minimizing respiratory depression and risks associated with anesthesia and analgesia.

REFERENCES

1. Caplan RA, Posner KL, Ward RJ, Cheney FW: Adverse respiratory events in anesthesia: a closed claims analysis. Anesthesiology 1990; 72:828-33
2. Rekling JC, Feldman JL: Pre-Botzinger complex and pacemaker neurons: hypothesized site and kernel for respiratory rhythm generation. Ann Rev Physiol 1998; 60:385-405

3. Nattie EE: Central Chemoreception, Regulation of Breathing, second Edition. Dempsey JA, Pack AI, eds. New York, Marcel Dekker, Inc. 1995, pp 473-510

4. Dahan A, Berkenbosch A: Ventilatory response to carbon dioxide. [letter; comment] Br J Anaesth 1996; 76:747-8

5. Jacobi MS, Patil CP, Sunders KB: Transient, steady-state, and rebreathing responses to carbon dioxide in man, at rest and during light exercise. J Physiol 1989; 411:85-96

6. Bourke DL, Warley A: The steady-state and rebreathing methods compared during morphine administration in humans. J Physiol (Lon) 1989; 419:509-17

7. Dahan A, Berkenbosch A, DeGeode J, Olievier ICW, Bovill JG: On a pseudo-rebreathing technique to assess the ventilatory sensitivity to carbon dioxide in man. J Physiol 1990; 423:615-29

8. Linton RAF, Poole-Wilson PA, Davies RJ, Cameron IR: A comparison of the ventilatory response to carbon dioxide by steady-state and rebreathing methods during metabolic acidosis and alkalosis. Clin Sci and Molec Med 1973; 45:239-49

9. Berkenbosch A, Bovill JG, Dahan A, DeGeode J, Olievier ICW: The ventilatory CO_2 sensitivities from Read's rebreathing method and the steady-state method are not equal in man. J Physiol 1989; 411:367-77

10. Johnson A, Löfström JB: A new method for studying the ventilatory response in patients. Acta Anaesthesiol Scan 1990; 34:440-6

11. Weil JV, McCullough RE, Kline JS, Sodal IE: Diminished ventilatory response to hypoxia and hypercapnia after morphine in normal man. NEJM 1975; 292:1103-8

12. Rebuck AS, Campbell EJM: A clinical method for assessing the ventilatory response to hypoxia. Amer Rev Resp Dis 1974; 109:345-50

13. Easton PA, Slykerman LJ, Anthonisen NR: Recovery of the ventilatory response to hypoxia in normal adults. J Appl Physiol 1988; 64:521-8

14. Easton PA, Anthonisen NR: Carbon dioxide effects on the ventilatory response to sustained hypoxia. J Appl Physiol 1988; 64:1451-6

15. Tatsumi K, Pickett CK, Weil JV: Attenuated carotid body hypoxic sensitivity after prolonged hypoxic exposure. J Appl Physico 1991; 70:748-55

16. Bailey PL, Andriano KP, Goldman M, Stanley TH, Pace NL: Variability of the respiratory response to diazepam. Anesthesiology 1986; 64:460-5

17. Bailey PL, Pace NL, Ashburn MA, Moll JWB, East KA, Stanley TH: Frequent hypoxemia and apnea after sedation with midazolam and fentanyl. Anesthesiology 1990; 73:826-30

18. Temp JA, Henson LC, Ward DS: Effect of a subanesthetic minimum alveolar concentration of isoflurane on two tests of the hypoxic ventilatory response. Anesthesiology 1994; 80:739-50

19. Dahan A, van den Elsen M, Berkenbosch A, DeGoede J, Olievier IC, van Kleef JW, Bovill JG: Effects of subanesthetic halothane on the ventilatory responses to hypercapnia and acute hypoxia in healthy volunteers. Anesthesiology 1994; 80:727-38

20. Robotham JL: Do low-dose inhalational anesthetic agents alter ventilatory control? [editorial; comment] [see comments] Anesthesiology 1994; 80:723-6

21. Dahan A, Sarton E, van den Elsen M, van Kleef J, Teppema L, Berkenbosch A: Ventilatory response to hypoxia in humans. Anesthesiology 1996; 85:60-8

22. Flórez J, Hurlé MA: Opioids in respiration and vomiting, Opioids II - Handbook of experimental pharmacology. Herz A. Berlin, ed. Springer-Verlag, 1993, pp 263-92

23. Shook JE, Watkins WD, Camporesi EM: Differential roles of opioid receptors in respiration, respiratory disease, and opiate-induced respiratory depression. Am Rev Respir Dis 1990; 142:895-909

24. Wamsley JK: Opioid receptors: autoradiography. Pharmacol Rev 1983; 35:69-83

25. Santiago TV, Edelman NH: Opioids and breathing. J Appl Physiol 1985; 59:1675-85

26. Hickey RF, Severinghaus JW: Regulation of breathing: Drug effects, Lung Biology in Health and Disease. Hornbein T., ed. New York, Marcel Dekker, 1981, pp 1251-98

27. Ngai SH: Effects of morphine and meperidine on the central respiratory mechanisms in the cat, the action of levallorphan in antagonizing these effects. J Pharmacol Exp Ther 1961; 131:91-9

28. Tabatabai M, Kitahata LM, Collins JG: Disruption of the rhythmic activity of the medullary inspiratory neurons and phrenic nerve by fentanyl and reversal with nalbuphine. Anesthesiology 1989; 70:489-95

29. Chen S-W, Maguire PA, Daview MF, Beety MF, Loew GH: Evidence for m_1-opioid receptor involvement in fentanyl-mediated respiratory depression. Euro J Pharmacol 1996; 312:241-4

30. Kryger MH, Yacoub 0, Dosman J, Macklem PT, Anthonisen NR: Effect of meperidine on occlusion pressure responses to hypercapnia and hypoxia with and without external inspiratory resistance. Am Rev Respir Dis 1976; 114:333-40

31. Weil JV, Byrne-Quinn E, Sodal IE, Friesen WO, Underhill B, Filley GF, Grover RF: Hypoxic ventilatory drive in normal man. J Clin Investigation 1970; 49:1061-72

32. Cartwright P, Prys-Roberts C, Gill K, Dye A, Stafford M, Gray A: Ventilatory depression related to plasma fentanyl concentrations

during and after anesthesia in humans. Anesth Analg 1983; 62:966-74

33. Bailey PL, Rhondeau S, Schafer PG, Lu JK, Timmins BS, Foster W, Pace NL, Stanley TH: Dose-response pharmacology of intrathecal morphine in human volunteers. Anesthesiology 1993; 79:49-59

34. Drummond GB: Comparison of decreases in ventilation caused by enflurane and fentanyl during anesthesia. Br J Anaesth 1983; 55:825-35

35. Berkowitz BA, Ngai SH, Yang JC, Hempstead J, Spector S: The disposition of morphine in surgical patients. Clin Pharmacol Ther 1975; 17:629-35

36. Nielsen CH, Camporesi EM, Bromage PR, Bukowski EM, Durant PAC: CO_2 sensitivity after epidural and IV morphine. Anesthesiology 1981; 55:A372

37. Downes JJ, Kemp RA, Lambertsen CJ: The magnitude and duration of respiratory depression due to fentanyl and meperidine in man. J Pharmacol Exp Therap 1967; 158:416-20

38. Bailey PL, Streisand JB, East KA, East TD, Isern S, Hansen TW, Posthuma FM, Rozendaal FW, Pace NL, Stanley TH: Differences in magnitude and duration of opioid-induced respiratory depression and analgesia with fentanyl and sufentanil. Anesth Analg 1990; 70:8-15

39. Holmes CM: Supplementation of general anaesthesia with narcotic analgesics. Br J Anaesth 1976; 48:907-13

40. Hug CC Jr, Murphy MR: Fentanyl disposition in cerebrospinal fluid and plasma and its relationship to ventilatory depression in the dog. Anesthesiology 1979; 50:342-9

41. Osei-Gyimah P, Archer S: Some 14-beta-substituted analogues of N-(cyclopropylmethyl) nor-morphine. J Med Chem 1981; 24:212

42. Shafer SL, Varvel JR: Pharmacokinetics, pharmacodynamics, and rational opioid selection. Anesthesiology 1991; 74:53-63

43. Cookson RF, Niemegeers CJE, Vanden Bussche G: The development of alfentanil. Br J Anaesth 1983; 55:147S-55S

44. Ausems ME, Hug Carl C J, Stanski DR, Burm AG: Plasma concentrations of alfentanil required to supplement nitrous oxide anesthesia for general surgery. Anesthesiology 1986; 65:362-73

45. Reed DJ, Kellog RH: Changes in respiratory response to CO_2 during natural sleep at sea level and at altitude. J Appl Physiol 1958; 13:325-30

46. Forrest WH, Bellville JW: The effect of sleep plus morphine on the respiratory response to carbon dioxide. Anesthesiology 1964; 25:137-41

47. Kurth CD: Postoperative arterial oxygen saturation: what to expect. Anesth Analg 1995; 80:1-3

48. Rosenberg-Adamsen S, Kehlet H, Dodds C, Resenberg J: Postoperative sleep disturbances: mechanisms and clinical implications. Br J Anaesth 1996; 76:552-9

49. Rigg JRA, Rondi P: Changes in rib cage and diaphragm contribution to ventilation after morphine. Anesthesiology 1981; 55:507-14
50. Longobardo GE, Gothe B, Goldman MD, Cherniak NS: Sleep apnea considered as a control system instability. Respir Physiol 1982; 50:311-33
51. Bailey PL, Wilbrink J, Zwanikken P, Pace NL, Stanley TH: Anesthetic induction with fentanyl. Anesth Analg 1985; 64:48
52. Foldes FF, Swerdlow M, Siker ES: Narcotics and narcotic antagonists. Springfield, IL, Charles C Thomas, 1964
53. Bentley JB, Borel JD, Nenad REJ, Gillespie TJ: Age and fentanyl pharmacokinetics. Anesth Analg 1982; 61:968-71
54. Arunasalam K, Davenport HT, Painter S, Jones JG: Ventilatory response to morphine in young and old subjects. Anaesthesia 1983; 38:529-33
55. Way WL, Costley EC, Way EL: Respiratory sensitivity of the newborn to meperidine and morphine. Clin Pharmacol Ther 1965; 6:454-61
56. Eckenhoff JE, Oech SR: The effects of narcotics and antagonists upon respiration and circulation in man. Clin Pharmacol Ther 1960; 1:483-524
57. Becker LD, Paulson BA, Miller RD, Severinghaus JW, Eger EI: Biphasic respiratory depression after fentanyl-droperidol or fentanyl alone used to supplement nitrous oxide anesthesia. Anesthesiology 1976; 44:291-6
58. Harper MH, Hickey RF, Cromwell TH, Linwood S: The magnitude and duration of respiratory depression produced by fentanyl and fentanyl plus droperidol in man. J Pharmacol Exp Ther 1976; 199:464-8
59. Bailey PL, Sperry RJ, Johnson GK, Eldredge SJ, East KA, East TD, Pace NL, Stanley TH: Respiratory effects of clonidine alone and combined with morphine, in humans. Anesthesiology 1991; 74:43-8
60. Furst SR, Weinger MB: Dexmedetomidine, a selective a_2-agonist, does not potentiate the cardiorespiratory depression of alfentanil in the rat. Anesthesiology 1990; 72:882-8
61. Tyler DC: Respiratory effects of pain in child after thoracotomy. Anesthesiology 1989; 70:873
62. Rawal N, Wattwil M: Respiratory depression after epidural morphine - an experimental and clinical study. Anesth Analg 1984; 63:8-14
63. Nishino T, Hiraga K, Fujisato M, Mizuguchi T, Honda Y: Breathing patterns during postoperative analgesia in patients after lower abdominal operations. Anesthesiology 1988; 69:967-72
64. Sarton E, Dahan A, Teppema L, van den Elsen M, Olofsen E, Berkenbosch A, van Kleef J: Acute pain and central nervous system arousal do not restore impaired hypoxic ventilatory response during sevoflurane sedation. Anesthesiology 1996; 85:295-303

65. Sarton E, Dahan A, Teppeman L, Berkenbosch A, van den Elsen M, van Kleef J: Influence of acute pain induced by activation of cutaneous nociceptors on ventilatory control. Anesthesiology 1997; 87:289-96

66. Pelligrino DA, Riegler FX, Albrecht RF: Ventilatory effects of fourth cerebroventricular infusions of morphine-6- or morphine-3-glucuronide in the awake dog. Anesthesiology 1989; 71:936-40

67. Peat SJ, Hanna MH, Woodham M, Knibb AA, Ponte J: Morphine-6-glucuronide: effects on ventilation in normal volunteers. Pain 1991; 45:101-4

68. Ainslie SG, Eisele JH, Corkill G: Fentanyl concentrations in brain and serum during respiratory acid-base changes in the dog. Anesthesiology 1979; 51:293-7

69. Beard K, Hershel J, Walker AM: Adverse respiratory events occurring in the recovery room after general anesthesia. Anesthesiology 1986; 64:269-72

70. Severinghaus JW, Kelleher JF: Recent developments in pulse oximetry. Anesthesiology 1992; 76:1018-38

71. Bailey PL: The use of opioids in anesthesia is not especially associated with nor predictive of postoperative hypoxemia. (Correspondence) Anesthesiology 1992; 77:1235

72. Catley DM, Thornton C, Jordan C, Lehane JR, Royston D, Jones JG: Pronounced episodic oxygen desaturation in the postoperative period: its association with ventilatory pattern and analgesic regimen. Anesthesiology 1985; 63:20-8

WHEN DOES THE INFANT MATURE PHARMACOLOGICALLY?

Dennis M. Fisher

INTRODUCTION

Two assumptions regarding the pharmacologic response of neonates to intravenous anesthetic drugs are common: first, that neonates are "sensitive" to these agents; and second, that recovery from these agents is slower compared to adults. Although these assumptions are sometimes correct, they are often untrue. In this session, I will review certain maturational changes in body structure and organ function during the neonatal period and infancy and examine how these changes alter the response of neonates and infants to intravenous anesthetics. For consistency, I use the term neonate for the full-term neonate less than 30 days, infant for the child aged 1-12 months, and child for children greater than one year of age.

MATURATIONAL CHANGES IN BODY COMPOSITION

The first year of life represents a period of rapid change in body composition. Most significant to the maturation in pharmacologic response are the changes in body water (particularly extracellular fluid volume) (1), the mass of the liver (2), and creation of fat stores (1, 3). The extracellular fluid volume (ECF) of the fetus represents 55% of body weight decreasing to 44% of body weight at term (1). During infancy, ECF decreases further, approaching the adult value (21-22%) by one year of age (1). This 2-3 fold change affects those drugs whose distribution is limited to extracellular water, particularly muscle relaxants. For example, we demonstrated that the *d*-tubocurarine's volume of distribution at steady-state is greatest in neonates and greater in infants than in children and

T. H. Stanley and T. D. Egan (eds.), Anesthesia for the New Millennium, 49–54.
© *1999 Kluwer Academic Publishers.*

adults (4). Similar findings were reported for vecuronium and atracurium (5, 6). As a result, when these drugs are administered based on weight (or lean body mass, as may be appropriate in adults), plasma concentration will be lower in younger patients.

Liver mass represents a larger percentage of body weight at birth than at subsequent periods (2). However, at birth, the large mass of the liver does not necessarily assure a large metabolic capacity — maturation of elimination pathways must also be considered. Once hepatic maturity is achieved (typically by one month of age; see below), the liver's large mass may permit high metabolic clearance in infants. For example, fentanyl's clearance is greatest during infancy.

At birth, fat stores are negligible, increasing markedly during the first year of life (1, 3). As a result, the distribution volume for fat-soluble drugs should be lower in the youngest patients. However, because volume of distribution at steady-state (Vss) is also a function of plasma protein binding, maturational changes in Vss for fat-soluble anesthetic drugs may be less evident.

A fourth factor that influences drug distribution and elimination is the concentration of plasma proteins. Although the specific relationship of plasma proteins to drug elimination is often quite complicated (and is important only when the drug is highly bound to one or more proteins), the concentration of plasma proteins is often lower in younger patients (7), and in some cases, the affinity of these proteins for drugs is lower than in adults (8). As a result, protein binding is generally lower in younger patients than in the mature patient.

MATURATIONAL CHANGES IN BODY FUNCTION

Just as the size/volume of various body compartments varies during the first year(s) of life, organ function also changes markedly during this period. Following the precipitous changes of the transitional circulation at birth, basal cardiac output is high during the first month of life, then decreases gradually during the first year of life. The high cardiac output during early periods results in rapid delivery of drugs to their site of action; hence, onset of most drugs should be hastened in the neonatal period. This rapid onset in infancy has been demonstrated for most muscle relaxants. Onset of effect for other drugs such as opioids has also been observed clinically although scientific confirmation is lacking.

A corollary of the high cardiac output is that hepatic blood flow should also be highest during the neonatal period; however, the complex relationship between the portal venous and hepatic arterial systems, coupled with the presence of blood flow through a patent ductus venosus, confounds this issue during the neonatal period (9, 10). Once the ductus venosus has closed (likely during the first week of life) and liver function matures, hepatic clearance of drugs highly extracted by the liver may actually be highest during infancy. This has been demonstrated for fentanyl (11).

Further confounding the liver's role in drug metabolism are the maturational states of the various hepatic metabolic pathways (about which relatively little is known in humans). Three elimination pathways exist — mixed function oxidases (cytochrome P450), conjugation (e.g., glucuronidation), and biliary excretion of intact drug. The first of these, the cytochrome P450 pathway, has been better studied in animals than in humans. Studies in human abortuses suggest that concentrations of P450 are low or absent in the fetus (12) and that maternal exposure to drugs that induce hepatic function have little effect on the fetus (13). In calves, activity of various cytochrome P450 isoenzymes is low at birth, increasing markedly, but at different rates, during the first month of life (14). For example, O-deethylase activity at one week of age exceeds mature values, whereas N-demethylase and O-demethylase activity remains immature at one week of age (14). For obvious reasons, comparable studies in humans are lacking.

Conjugation develops after birth. For example, conjugation of barbiturates to glucosides, absent at birth, develops during the first weeks of life (15), while morphine's conjugation to glucuronides develops after the first weeks of life (16, 17). Finally, little is know about biliary excretion of anesthetic drugs during the first weeks of life.

Renal function, as assessed by glomerular filtration, is low at birth, increasing markedly during the first year of life. For example, *d*-tubocurarine, whose predominant elimination pathway is via glomerular filtration, has low clearance at birth, reaching adult values at one year of age, (4) parallel to maturational changes in glomerular filtration rate (18).

Finally, the blood-brain barrier behaves differently in the neonate than in the older subject. Following its maturation, the blood-brain barrier limits passage of lipophobic substances into the brain. However, in the neonate it appears that this barrier is less well developed, permitting rapid passage of lipophobic substances into the brain. Lipophilic substances should not be affected by maturational changes in the blood-brain barrier, as they cross the intact barrier readily. This was proposed by Kupferberg and Way (19) as the explanation for the age-related changes in sensitivity in morphine. However, two recent studies from our laboratory challenge their findings. In the first study, Bragg et al. (20) examined the maturational changes in ventilatory depression in puppies aged 1 day to 1 month. Although k_{eo} (the rate constant for equilibration between plasma concentrations and effect) differed between morphine and fentanyl, it did not change with age for either drug. However, steady-state sensitivity to morphine changed approximately 100-fold during that maturational period whereas steady-state sensitivity to fentanyl changed only 4-fold (20). A second study by Luks et al. (21) examined the analgesic effects of these two drugs in a second group of similarly-aged puppies. Again, k_{eo} differed between drugs but did not vary with age. For both drugs, there were small (and parallel) maturational changes in steady-state sensitivity to the opioid. The findings from these two studies suggest an interesting explanation for reluctance of clinicians to give morphine to neonates. Whereas morphine-induced analgesia and ventilatory depression occur at similar concentrations in the mature humans or animal, the 1-day old develops morphine-induced ventilatory depression at concentrations less than those that induce analgesia. The occurrence of respiratory depression with analgesia minimizes the utility of morphine in younger animals and people. However, for fentanyl, maturational changes in analgesia and ventilatory depression are parallel so that doses that are ventilatory depressant also induce analgesia.

THE ANSWER (?)

Critical examination of the response of infants and children to intravenous anesthetics is often lacking. There are several reasons for this. First, performing control clinical trials is often difficult; obtaining blood samples, as is necessary for most pharmacokinetic/

pharmacodynamic studies, further complicates obtaining appropriate information in younger patients. Second, many investigators perform studies in infants and children, but not in adults, relying instead on published data for comparisons. When studies in adults are performed in different institutions and using different methodologies, it is often difficult to make age-related comparisons.

In the absence of adequate data, only limited conclusions can be drawn. First, most changes in body composition occur during the neonatal period and infancy; thus, maturational changes affecting drug distribution are largely complete by one year of age. Second, most of the changes in organ function, such as maturation of hepatic metabolic pathways and renal function, are similarly complete by one year of age; thus, drug elimination varies little after one year of age. A reasonable summary is that the response of the neonate and infant can be expected to differ from that of the adult, but that the child greater than one year of age differs relatively little from the adult.

REFERENCES

1. Friis-Hansen B: Body composition during growth. *In-vivo* measurements and biochemical data correlated to differential anatomical growth. Pediatrics 1971; 47: 264-74
2. Nayak NC, Ramalingaswami V: Normal structure, The Liver and Biliary System in Infants and Children. Edited by Chandra R. Edinburgh, Churchill Livingstone, 1979, pp 1-17
3. Petersen S, Gotfredsen A, Knudsen FU: Lean body mass in small for gestational age and appropriate for gestational age infants. J Pediatr 1988; 113: 886-9
4. Fisher DM, O'Keeffe C, Stanski DR, Cronnelly R, Miller RD, Gregory GA: Pharmacokinetics and pharmacodynamics of *d*-tubocurarine in infants, children, and adults. Anesthesiology 1982; 57: 203-8
5. Fisher DM, Castagnoli K, Miller RD: Vecuronium kinetics and dynamics in anesthetized infants and children. Clin Pharmacol Ther 1985; 37: 402-6
6. Fisher DM, Canfell PC, Spellman MJ, Miller RD: Pharmacokinetics and pharmacodynamics of atracurium in infants and children. Anesthesiology 1990; 73: 33-7
7. Notarianni LJ: Plasma protein binding of drugs in pregnancy and in neonates. Clin Pharmacokinet 1990; 18: 20-36
8. Brodersen R, Honore B: Drug binding properties of neonatal albumin. Acta Paediatr Scand 1989; 78: 342-6

54

9. Botti JJ, Edelstone DI, Caritis SN, Mueller-Heubach E: Portal venous blood flow distribution to liver and ductus venosus in newborn lambs. Am J Obstet Gynecol 1982; 144: 303-8
10. Edelstone DI, Rudolph AM, Heymann MA: Liver and ductus venosus blood flows in fetal lambs in utero. Circ Res 1978; 42: 426-33
11. Gauntlett IS, Fisher DM, Hertzka RE, Kuhls E, Spellman MJ, Rudolph C: Pharmacokinetics of fentanyl in neonatal humans and lambs: Effects of age. Anesthesiology 1988; 69: 683-7
12. Juchau MR, Chao ST, Omiecinski CJ: Drug metabolism by the human fetus. Clin Pharm 1980; 5: 320-39
13. Sereni F, Mandelli M, Principi N, Tognoni G, Pardi G, Morselli PL: Induction of drug metabolizing enzyme activities in the human fetus and in the newborn infant. Enzyme 1973; 15: 318-29
14. Shoaf SE, Schwark WS, Guard CL, Babish JG: The development of hepatic drug-metabolizing enzyme activity in the neonatal calf and its effect on drug disposition. Drug Metab Dispos 1987; 15: 676-81
15. Bhargava VO, Garrettson LK: Development of phenobarbital glucosidation in the human neonate. Dev Pharmacol Ther 1988; 11: 8-13
16. Bhat R, Chari G, Gulati A, Aldana O, Velamati R, Bhargava H: Pharmacokinetics of a single dose of morphine in preterm infants during the first week of life. J Pediatr 1990; 117: 477-81
17. Bhat R, Abu HM, Chari G, Gulati A: Morphine metabolism in acutely ill preterm newborn infants. J Pediatr 1992; 120: 795-9
18. Chantler C: Evaluation of laboratory and other methods of measuring renal function, Clinical Pediatric Nephrology. Edited by Lieberman E. Philadelphia, JB Lippincott, 1976, pp 515
19. Kupferberg HJ, Way EL: Pharmacologic basis for the increased sensitivity of the newborn rat to morphine. J Pharmacol Exp Ther 1963; 141: 105-12
20. Bragg P, Zwass MS, Lau M, Fisher DM: Opioid pharmacodynamics in neonatal dogs: differences between morphine and fentanyl. J Appl Physiol 1995; 79: 1519-24
21. Luks AM, Zwass MS, Brown RC, Lau M, Chari G, Fisher DM: Opioid-induced analgesia in neonatal dogs: pharmacodynamic differences between morphine and fentanyl. J Pharmacol Exp Ther 1998; 284: 136-41

BRAIN IMAGING FOR ELUCIDATING MECHANISMS OF ANESTHESIA

Pierre Fiset

Positron Emission Tomography (PET) and functional Magnetic Resonance Imaging (fMRI) allow researchers to study brain function in vivo. Those techniques are used to refine our understanding of the nature of anesthetic effects as well as of the influence of anesthetic drugs on sensory and pain transmission.

HOW THEY WORK

PET

PET uses a combination of scintigraphic and computerized tomography techniques. A biological compound labeled with a radioactive tracer (^{11}C, ^{13}N, ^{15}O, ^{18}F) is injected into a subject so that its distribution in the target tissue can be determined. Once in the tissue, the isotope emits a positron that collides with and annihilates a neighboring electron to emit energy in the form of two g rays traveling in opposite direction. The scanner is made of a circumferential ring of scintillation detectors which look for coincidence events, i.e., two g ray interactions that occur almost simultaneously on opposite sides of the head. After a series of transformations and correction procedures, a cross-sectional image of the detected counts is created. This image is then "stretched" into a stereotaxic space to allow standardization of anatomical location and inter-subject comparisons. An MRI scan is always obtained in a subsequent session to allow precise anatomical localization of brain structures.

Depending on the information desired, a variety of compounds can be labeled. For functional brain studies, ^{15}O labeled water is often used for determination of regional Cerebral Blood Flow (rCBF) based on the assumption that changes in rCBF are coupled with those of neuronal

T. H. Stanley and T. D. Egan (eds.), Anesthesia for the New Millennium, 55–61.

activity. Cerebral metabolic rate studies are performed with labeled glucose or oxygen. It is also possible to study neurotransmission by looking at the displacement of a labeled ligand from its binding sites (1). For example, ^{11}C benztropine, an M_1 and M_2 non-specific antagonist, is used by our group to study cholinergic muscarinic transmission under anesthesia. PET has been used for more than a decade for localization of human cognitive operations (2).

The basis of PET studies is to submit a group of individuals to a series of different conditions and to statistically compare the images to determine the physiologic changes induced by a given condition. Examples of conditions are: increasingly painful stimuli, increasing levels of drug sedation, and a mixture of painful stimuli at increasing levels of sedation. A comparison between conditions is made by using a voxel-based analysis that will result in a statistical map of the magnitude of changes in any region of the brain. For blood flow studies, comparisons are made using a subtraction technique (a given stimulus vs no stimulus) or a regression technique (influence of the level of sedation on rCBF). Complex time dependent analyses are made to determine receptor occupancy in ligand studies.

fMRI

fMRI uses a different principle. Again, the basis of the studies is to compare changes in brain activation induced between conditions in a strictly controlled experimental environment, but there is no need for radioactive tracers, and the temporal and spatial resolutions are much better than with PET.

During an MRI scan, the magnetic fields from hydrogen nuclei of water molecules orient themselves along the strong magnetic field of the scanner. Radio frequency pulses are sent to disturb this orientation. The resulting realignment causes the emission of a radio frequency signal that can be detected by a receiver coil (3).

In brain regions activated during neuronal stimulation, the signal is increased by a change in the ratio of deoxyhemoglobin. During neuronal activity, local metabolism increases and local blood flow increases more than in proportion for the demand, inducing a paradoxical decrease in the ratio of deoxyhemoglobin. It is the resulting "blood oxygen level dependent" (BOLD) signal that constitutes the basis of fMRI (4).

BRAIN IMAGING AND ANESTHESIA

Brain imaging offers unique possibilities for improving our knowledge of anesthetic effects. Anesthesia induces a host of dose-specific and controllable changes in CNS function. Our knowledge of pharmacology and the availability of powerful tools to achieve and maintain stable drug concentrations allow us to use anesthetic drugs as modulators of consciousness. Stable levels, or conditions in the brain imaging vocabulary, can be obtained that correspond to specific levels of sedation. The dose specific changes in brain activity can be measured, and the neurophysiological correlates of the regional changes can be explored. Brain imaging allows us to have a systems approach to the investigation of mechanisms of anesthesia. It is based on the premise that anesthetic drugs possibly have a dose-dependent effect on specific neural systems.

Potential target areas for anesthetic drug effects are the reticular-thalamic activating system, sensory and pain pathways, associative areas and areas related to memory. Of course, the experimental design has to be carefully controlled so that the condition obtained correlates with the function to investigate. Most studies are done on volunteers, and extreme ethical and security criteria are to be met.

REVIEW OF EXISTING LITERATURE

Pet Studies

Alkire et al. studied propofol anesthesia in human volunteers using ^{18}fluorodeoxyglucose (FDG) (5). Two conditions were obtained: awake and unconscious (mean propofol concentration of 3.5 ±0.6 mg·ml^{-1}). They reported that propofol produced a global metabolic depression on the human central nervous system, more pronounced in the cortical than sub-cortical areas. Regional cortical differences were not prominent. The same group studied isoflurane-induced unconsciousness in human volunteers (6) submitted to two conditions: awake and isoflurane (end-tidal 0.5 ± 0.1%). They report a uniform decrease in cerebral glucose metabolism with no specific regional changes.

Using ^{15}O labeled water, the Pittsburgh group has reported regional effects after administration of 20% Nitrous oxide alone (7) and during noxious heat stimuli (8). The pattern and localization of change in neuronal activation was coherent with the behavioral effects of N2O. N2O decreased activation in the areas typically related to pain perception (thalamus, supplementary motor area and anterior cingulate) while the subjects experienced a decrease in subjective pain experience.

The same group studied the effects of fentanyl alone (9) and coupled with the administration of tonic painful heat (10). They report a fentanyl-induced increase in rCBF in areas of the CNS responsive to nociceptive stimuli and a decrease in other areas. This complex pattern of effects makes their data on pain modulation difficult to interpret. Additionally, the methodology for fentanyl dosage and administration as well as the timing of scan acquisition to peak drug effect are questionable.

Finally, Veselis et al. (11) carefully studied the effects of midazolam using ^{15}H2O. They report dose-related changes in rCBF in brain regions associated with the normal functioning of arousal, attention, and memory.

fMRI Studies

This investigational technique being relatively newer than PET, little research has been done on anesthetic action using fMRI. One study was published by Antognini et al. (12) on the effect of isoflurane on tactile and pain stimulation. Results are difficult to interpret because the fMRI signal is affected by blood flow, and no correction can be made for the vasodilation effect of isoflurane.

EFFECTS OF PROPOFOL

In 1996, our group started to study the effects of propofol on the CNS using PET. In a first study, we have determined the effect of different levels of propofol sedation, from light sedation to unconsciousness, on rCBF using ^{15}H2O (13). We found a significant decrease in rCBF of the thalamus, the orbito-frontal cortices, and a large area of the medial parieto-occipital cortex extending bilaterally to the parietooccipital sulcus area. These anatomical sites are involved in the control of consciousness and in various integrative and associative tasks. These results support the hypothesis that propofol has regional effects and that certain brain structures might have a specific sensitivity to anesthetic effect. If these results are confirmed, the notion that precise neural networks are involved in the maintenance of anesthetic effects should help guiding research on cellular and molecular mechanisms of anesthesia.

The neural pathways for conducting and perceiving pain and vibro-tactile stimulation are well known, and their activation following a stimulus can be clearly and accurately shown using PET (14,15). It is the very nature of anesthesia to alter the perception of external stimuli, thus allowing the performance of noxious operations, but very little is known on the exact mechanism by which such a disruption of neural conduction happens. Is the stimulus blocked at the level of the dorsal horn, the thalamus, the primary or secondary sensory cortex? Are we only modulating the associative and affective functions related to pain perception? Do these areas of the CNS show a dose-dependent sensitivity to anesthetics?

We have conducted a study on the influence of the level of propofol sedation on vibro-tactile stimulation (16). Volunteers were submitted to increasing target concentrations of propofol and presented with standardized vibratory stimuli. We found a significant decrease in activation of the primary and secondary sensory cortex as well as the thalamus at very low sedative doses of propofol (0.5 mg·ml^{-1}). A more profound effect is seen at higher levels of sedation, with an almost complete abolition of activation when pharmacological unconsciousness is reached. This suggests that even when a patient is only mildly sedated, a rather significant effect on neuronal conduction might explain a relative indifference to external tactile stimuli.

PET allowed us to explore another aspect of anesthetic action related to neurotransmission. There are reports in the literature of reversal of anesthetic effects with physostigmine, an anticholinesterase drug that crosses the blood-brain barrier. In fact Antilirium® has been used for years to "speed up awakening." It is also common knowledge that scopolamine, an antimuscarinic drug that also crosses the blood-brain barrier, induces sedation and potentiates anesthetic effect. These facts, coupled with the extensive knowledge on the modulatory effect of the central cholinergic system on sleep-wake states, suggest that the central muscarinic system has a role to play in the generation of anesthetic effect. We have used a nonspecific M1 and M2 antagonist, ^{11}C-Benztropine, to study muscarinic receptor occupancy during propofol unconsciousness.

CONCLUSION

Brain imaging is a window on the working brain. It offers tremendous possibilities for understanding the neural processes involved in all aspects of consciousness. Anesthesiologists possess the pharmacological knowledge and clinical skills that allow them to modulate the conscious behavior in a safe and controlled fashion, putting them in a position to make major contributions to the field of neuroscience.

BIBLIOGRAPHY

1. Saha GB, MacIntyre WJ, Go RT: Radiopharmaceuticals for brain imaging. Seminars in Nuclear Medicine 24:324-349, 1994
2. Posner MI, Petersen SE, Fox PT, Raichle ME: Localization of cognitive operations in the human brain. Science 240:1627-1631, 1988
3. Le Bihan D, Jezzard P, Haxby J, Sadato N, Rueckert L, Mattay V: Functional magnetic resonance imaging of the brain. Annals of Internal Medicine 122:296-303, 1995
4. Ogawa S, Tank DW, Menon R, Ellermann JM, Kim S-G, Merkle H, Ugurbil K: Intrinsic signal changes accompanying sensory stimulation: functional brain mapping with magnetic resonance imaging. Proc Natl Acad Sci 89:5951-5955, 1992
5. Alkire MT, Haier RJ, Barker SJ, Shah NK, Wu JC, Kao J: Cerebral metabolism during propofol anesthesia in humans studied with positron emission tomography. Anesthesiology 82:393-403, 1995
6. Alkire MT, Haler RJ, Shah NK, Anderson CT: Positron emission tomography study of regional cerebral metabolism in humans during isoflurane anesthesia. Anesthesiology 86:549-557, 1997
7. Gyulai FE, Firestone LL, Mintum MA, Winter PM: In Vivo imaging of human limbic responses to nitrous oxide inhalation. Anesth Analg 83:291-298, 1996
8. Gyulai FE, Firestone LL, Mintum MA, Winter PM: In vivo imaging of nitrous oxide-induced changes in cerebral activation during noxious heat stimuli. Anesthesiology 86:538-548, 1997
9. Firestone LL, Gyulai F, Mintun M, Adler LJ, Urso K, Winter PM: Human brain activity response to fentanyl imaged by positron emission tomography. Anesth Analg 82:1247-1251, 1996

10. Adler LJ, Gyulai FE, Diehl DJ, Mintum MA, Winter PM, Firestone LL: Regional brain activity changes associated with fentanyl analgesia elucidated by positron emission tomography. Anesth Analg 84:120-126, 1997

11. Veselis RA, Reinsel RA, Beattie BJ, Mawlawi OR, Feshchenko VA, DiResta GR, Larson SM, Blasberg RG: Midazolam changes cerebral blood flow in discrete brain regions. Anesthesiology 87:1106-1117, 1997

12. Antognini JF, Buonocore MH, Disbrow EA, Carsten E: Isoflurane anesthesia blunts cerebral responses to noxious and innocuous stimuli: a fMRI study. Life Sciences 61:349-354, 1997

13. Fiset P, Paus T, Daloze T, Plourde G, Hajj-Ali N, Evans A: Effect of propofol-induced anesthesia on regional cerebral blood-flow: a positron emission tomography study. Society for Neuroscience 22:357.111996(Abstract)

14. Coghill RC, Talbot JD, Evans AC, Meyer E, Gjedde A, Bushnell MC, Duncan GH: Distributed processing of pain and vibration by the human brain. Journal of Neuroscience 14:4095-4108, 1994

15. Talbot JD, Marret S, Evans AC, Meyer E, Bushnell MC, Duncan GH: Multiple representations of pain in human cerebral cortex. Science 251:1355-1357, 1991

16. Fiset P, Bonhomme V, Meuret P, Paus T, Plourde G, Backman SB, Bushnell C, Evans AC: Effects of Propofol on Regional Cerebral Blood Flow during Vibrotactile Stimulation in Man: A Positron Emission Tomography (PET) Study. Society for Neuroscience, 23: 398.14, 1997

IS PHARMACOKINETICS RELEVANT?

Dennis M. Fisher

During recent decades, the availability of assays to measure drug concentrations has resulted in a proliferation of pharmacokinetic studies. On occasion these studies provide tremendous insight into clinical problems. In this session, I will review some basic principles and study designs of pharmacokinetic and pharmacodynamic modeling and explain how these principles can facilitate clinical practice.

At its simplest, pharmacokinetics might require only a single value of drug concentration (typically measured in plasma). For example, if weight-normalized mivacurium infusion requirements are larger in children than in adults, does this result from maturational changes in pharmacokinetics (mivacurium's distribution and/or elimination characteristics) or pharmacodynamics (sensitivity of the neuromuscular junction)? If mivacurium were infused until twitch was stably depressed 50% (or 90% or 95%), a single plasma concentration value (Cp) might suffice to answer the question. First, comparison of infusion rates between the two groups would confirm the clinical observation. Second, comparison of the Cp values depressing twitch tension 50% (C_{50}) would inform about relative sensitivity. Finally, plasma clearance (Cl, determined as the ratio of infusion rate to Cp) could be compared. This simple study would confirm differences in dose requirements and provide insight into the origin of these differences.

Most pharmacokinetic studies are not performed at steady state so that more than one sample is typically obtained. Vecuronium's 25-75% recovery time being slower in infants than in children implies that its plasma concentration decreases more slowly in younger patients. If vecuronium concentrations were measured after a bolus dose (or a more

T. H. Stanley and T. D. Egan (eds.), Anesthesia for the New Millennium, 63–70.
© *1999 Kluwer Academic Publishers.*

complicated dosing regimen), one could determine the usual pharmacokinetic parameters. In this instance, Cl is similar in these two age groups (1). However, volume of distribution at steady state is larger in younger patients (presumably because vecuronium distributes into extracellular fluid, the volume of which decreases markedly during the first year of life), explaining the slower decrease in plasma concentrations of vecuronium. Again, we start with an observation and then use pharmacokinetic/pharmacodynamic modeling to explore that observation. If the results of the pharmacokinetic/pharmacodynamic study are consistent with our observation, we assume that the study has provided insight into the observation, i.e., it is clinically relevant.

A third approach extends the modeling to examine both pharmacokinetics, pharmacodynamics, and the rate of equilibration between plasma and effect site (e.g., the brain, the neuromuscular junction, etc.). We have all observed that morphine's onset is typically slow (10-15 minutes) and its duration long. In contrast, fentanyl's onset is always fast and its duration varies from short to long depending on dose. How can these observations be explained? Interestingly, the pharmacokinetic characteristics of the two drugs are quite similar, with Cl of 15 ml/kg/min and volume of distribution at steady state (Vss) of 4 L/kg; thus, pharmacokinetics does not explain differences between the two drugs. Steady state plasma concentrations that are effective (defined by analgesia, depression of ventilation, or some other measure) differ between the two drugs, thereby explaining the large difference in dose requirements between the drugs but still not explaining differences in time course. The picture is completed with measurements of the rate of equilibration between blood and brain: fentanyl equilibrates more rapidly than does morphine. This presumably results from morphine being water soluble, thereby entering and exiting the brain slowly, limiting its onset and offset. In contrast, fentanyl, being lipid soluble, enters and exiting the brain rapidly so its onset is always fast. The difference in offset of the two drugs can also be explained by the rate of equilibration — opioid effect dissipates as the brain concentration decreases to less than a threshold value. With a small fentanyl dose, this occurs rapidly during the initial rapid distribution phase; with larger doses, brain concentrations also decrease rapidly but remain above the threshold value for longer periods.

In contrast, morphine leaves the effect site slowly and cannot "take advantage" of its initial rapid distribution to facilitate recovery. The rate at which plasma and brain (effect site) concentrations equilibrate acquired the name k_{eo} based on Sheiner's seminal work with muscle relaxants (2). Thus, we can explain the difference between morphine and fentanyl not on their pharmacokinetic or steady state pharmacodynamic characteristics but rather on this rate of equilibration between blood and effect site.

The final approach to pharmacokinetic/pharmacodynamic modeling that I will discuss involves the concept of relevant half-life. Because our practice limits drug administration to brief periods (in contrast to chronic oral administration in most fields of medicine), we have little interest in the "late" pharmacokinetics of most drugs. For example, of what benefit is information regarding the elimination half-life of thiopental (12-24 hours) when the effects of a usual bolus dose dissipate in 10 minutes? A similar comment applies to propofol during anesthesia. Despite the lack of relevance of terminal half-life, the pharmacokinetic term in which most people are interested is half-life, and typically terminal half-life. There are various problems with the interpretation of half-lives. First, these values are extremely sensitive to study design. For example, VanderVeen and Bencini (3) reported that vecuronium's elimination half-life was 31 minutes while Fahey et al. (4) reported a value of 80 minutes. These two investigators used different assays with markedly different limits of detection, permitting drug identification for different periods of time. Unless the plasma concentration versus time curve has entered a log-linear phase, elimination half-life increases continuously with increasing sampling duration. The limitations of distribution half-life can be understood by considering the factors that influence our ability to accurately describe the rapid initial decline in plasma concentrations after bolus dosing. First, consider the differences between arterial and venous concentrations — venous values are smaller than arterial values during the initial phase, approaching and then eventually exceeding arterial concentrations. Second, consider what happens if the first sample is obtained at 1 minute versus 5 minutes — not obtaining early samples will not provide accurate information about the rapid changes occurring during the early distribution phase.

Recognizing marked limitations of many of the half-lives we commonly report has led to a change of philosophy. One global half-life — mean residence time — is defined as the ratio of Vss to Cl and represents the average time that a molecule spends within the body. This value first appeared in the anesthesia literature approximately 10 years ago with the intent of providing an "average" half-life, less affected by certain study design issues. In recent years an even "better" (i.e., more clinically relevant) half-life has been proposed. Hughes et al. (5) introduced the term "context sensitive half-time." Consider that a drug is infused at a constant rate for a period of time, then the infusion terminated. Context sensitive half-time is the time that it takes for Cp to decrease two-fold immediately after that infusion regimen (i.e., in that context). With brief infusions, rapid distribution dominates the decrease in plasma concentration; with lengthier infusions, the decrease in Cp is governed by elimination. Although relatively few drugs are given by infusion, the concept is relevant to the common regimen of repeat bolus administration.

Let us contrast these "clinically relevant" studies to other approaches to pharmacokinetics. Astute clinicians have observed that patients with renal failure are "sensitive" to the effects of morphine and assumed that the pharmacokinetics of morphine were altered by renal failure. Initial studies failed to find an effect of renal function on the pharmacokinetics of morphine. One might interpret these findings as questioning the clinical observation regarding the greater effects of morphine in patients with renal failure. However, I argue that when a consistent clinical observation is refuted by pharmacokinetic data, the critical reader should question the study rather than the observation! In fact, it was subsequently realized that a potent metabolite of morphine (morphine 6-glucuronide) is excreted by the kidneys and accumulates in patients with renal failure (6), thereby explaining the clinical observation.

When a new drug is undergoing clinical evaluation or use of a drug is to be extended to children, someone might determine its pharmacokinetics. These pharmacokinetic parameters might permit design of a drug administration regimen such as CACI (computer-assisted continuous infusions) targeting specific Cp values. However, in the absence of data regarding desired plasma (and effect site) concentrations, it is not useful to administer drugs to target concentrations. Thus, appropriate pharmacodynamic modeling is necessary to make the pharmacokinetic data useful. For example, if the only maturational change in the pharmacokinetics of ondansetron is that Cl is larger in children than in adults, will dose requirements be larger in children than in adults? Consider two scenarios. If sensitivity were the same in children and adults, then the larger Cl in younger patients might result in larger (or more frequent) dose requirements. However, if children demonstrated the same effect at lower Cp values, dose requirements might not vary with age. Another consideration is whether the effect of the drug is related temporally to the plasma concentration, in which case a decrease in brain concentrations should predict recurrence of vomiting. In contrast, the drug may reset the vomiting center, an effect that persists well after drug is gone from plasma. If the pharmacodynamic model is unknown, pharmacokinetic data are of limited utility: if the drug is "hit-and-run," there is no need to target constant Cp values.

There are other issues regarding the utility of pharmacokinetic data to design drug administration regimens. First, if there are active metabolites, the "effective" concentration is a function of the concentration of the parent compound and metabolite. Second, CACI is only useful if a drug equilibrates rapidly with the effect site. For example, CACI administration of morphine would maintain a constant plasma and brain concentration. However, intermittent boluses might maintain an equally constant brain concentration despite significant fluctuations in Cp values. Thus, fancy infusion regimens are wasted for morphine. In contrast, because fentanyl equilibrates rapidly between plasma and brain, both plasma and brain concentrations will fluctuate with repeated bolus dosing. Third, we need information regarding the specific kinetics and dynamics in the target population. If children differ markedly from adults in their pharmacokinetic and pharmacodynamic characteristics, it would be of no value to use data from adults to administer that drug to children.

The data presented thus far offer a cynical viewpoint that some reports of pharmacokinetics of anesthetic drugs provide little insight, i.e., they are not clinically relevant. In contrast, a small number of pharmacokinetic studies have provided tremendous insight. For example, Stanski's work on thiopental (7,8) has provided an understanding of why elderly people have a pronounced response to small doses of thiopental — although there is no difference in inherent brain sensitivity, age-related changes in distributional clearance result in the brain of elderly people "seeing" larger concentrations of the drug. Studies by Vuyk et al. (9,10) of the interaction of alfentanil and propofol provide insights into the interactions of these two drugs. Our own studies of muscle relaxants explain why dose requirements for these drugs are minimally affected by age but recovery from the effects of dTc and vecuronium (and to a lesser extent atracurium) are prolonged in infants (1,11,12). Our observation that infants 3-12 months of age "gobble" fentanyl is supported by our finding that clearance is largest in that age (13), presumably a result of a large liver mass and hepatic maturity at that age. Finally, a recent study examining the pharmacokinetics and ventilatory pharmacodynamics of fentanyl and morphine in neonatal dogs provides insight into the differences between these drugs (14). First, fentanyl equilibrates between brain and blood more rapidly than morphine, consistent with its more rapid onset. Second, morphine's sensitivity changes markedly during the first month of life, consistent with the numerous observations that neonates are "sensitive" to its effects. Although similar sensitivity in neonates is attributed to fentanyl, no clinical data support this claim. In addition, our clinical experience suggests that fentanyl dose requirements vary minimally during the first month of life. This is supported by the finding that neither sensitivity nor blood-brain barrier equilibration rates change with maturation. Thus, the maturational changes for morphine and fentanyl differ quite markedly.

Where does this leave the investigator with a new drug and an assay to measure that drug? I contend that a pharmacokinetic study that is not hypothesis-driven, lacks an appropriate control group, and lacks a pharmacodynamic component provides little insight into the drug's behavior, i.e., it is not clinically relevant. Studies that are clinically relevant are more difficult to perform but provide important information that guides our practice. A different example involves muscle relaxants, drugs for which we have an excellent understanding of the pharmacokinetic and pharmacodynamic models and for which there is great similarity between drugs. In general, if a new drug is expected to behave like the old drug, then simple pharmacokinetic studies might be useful. For example, knowing that active metabolites are minimally important with single doses of most relaxants, we need not consider metabolites in single dose studies. Yet, if a new relaxant that is extensively metabolized to an active compound became available, we would need to revise our models to incorporate this feature. Another example is mivacurium, a drug with three stereoisomers, two of which are potent, have different pharmacokinetic characteristics, and whose relatively potency in humans is unknown. Any pharmacokinetic model of this drug that does not account for its unique features will invariably be incorrect.

Where does that leave the clinician? Unfortunately, our journals are cluttered with pharmacokinetic studies in which the investigators have "an assay in search of a question" (I admit to having published some of these studies). These studies provide little insight. Fewer studies actually increase our understanding of our clinical practice. Hopefully the clinician can distinguish between the chaff and the wheat.

REFERENCES

1. Fisher DM, Castagnoli K, Miller RD: Vecuronium kinetics and dynamics in anesthetized infants and children. Clin Pharmacol Ther 1985; 37:402-6
2. Sheiner LB, Stanski DR, Vozeh S, Miller RD, Ham J: Simultaneous modeling of pharmacokinetics and pharmacodynamics: Application to d-tubocurarine. Clin Pharmacol Ther 1979; 25:358-71
3. VanderVeen F, Bencini A: Pharmacokinetics and pharmaco-dynamics of org nc45 in man. Br J Anaesth 1980; 52:37S-41S
4. Fahey MR, Morris RB, Miller RD, Nguyen T-L, Upton RA: Pharmacokinetics of Org NC45 (Norcuron) in patients with and without renal failure. Br J Anaesth 1981; 53:1049-53
5. Hughes MA, Glass PS, Jacobs JR: Context-sensitive half-time in multicompartment pharmacokinetic models for intravenous anesthetic drugs. Anesthesiology 1992; 76:334-41
6. Chauvin M, Sandouk P, Scherrmann JM, Farinotti R, Strumza P, Duvaldestin P: Morphine pharmacokinetics in renal failure. Anesthesiology 1987; 66:327-31
7. Homer TD, Stanski DR: The effect of increasing age on thiopental disposition and anesthetic requirement. Anesthesiology 1985; 62:714-24
8. Stanski DR, Maitre PO: Population pharmacokinetics and pharmacodynamics of thiopental: the effect of age revisited. Anesthesiology 1990; 72:412-22

70

9. Vuyk J, Hennis PJ, Burm AG, de Voogt JW, Spierdijk J: Comparison of midazolam and propofol in combination with alfentanil for total intravenous anesthesia. Anesth Analg 1990; 71:645-50

10. Vuyk J, Lim T, Engbers FH, Burm AG, Vletter AA, Bovill JG: Pharmacodynamics of alfentanil as a supplement to propofol or nitrous oxide for lower abdominal surgery in female patients. Anesthesiology 1993; 78:1036-45

11. Fisher DM, O'Keeffe C, Stanski DR, Cronnelly R, Miller RD, Gregory GA: Pharmacokinetics and pharmacodynamics of d-tubocurarine in infants, children, and adults. Anesthesiology 1982; 57:203-8

12. Fisher DM, Canfell PC, Spellman MJ, Miller RD: Pharmacokinetics and pharmacodynamics of atracurium in infants and children. Anesthesiology 1990; 73:33-7

13. Singleton MA, Rosen JI, Fisher DM: Plasma concentrations of fentanyl in infants, children and adults. Can J Anaesth 1987; 34:152-5

14. Bragg P, Fisher DM, Shi J, Donati F, Meistelman C, Lau M, Sheiner LB: Comparison of twitch depression of the adductor pollicis and the respiratory muscles. Pharmacodynamic modeling without plasma concentrations. Anesthesiology 1994; 80:310-9

PHYSIOLOGIC VS. PHARMACOLOGIC SLEEP

Pierre Fiset

Anesthesiologists are in a very privileged position to observe altered states of consciousness. On a daily basis, they use pharmacological compounds to modulate CNS responses to noxious stimuli. This is achieved in a very controlled fashion, the experienced clinician being able to maintain precise levels of sedation or depth of anesthesia. The complex neuronal network on which we act to alter consciousness has been extensively studied in the second half of this century. In fact, it is pertinent for the anesthesiologist to realize that natural sleep, another state of altered consciousness, does not occur by a passive mechanism of loss of wakefulness but rather, like anesthesia, by an active process. Sleep and anesthesia are not only conceptually related, they also share a variety of similar electrophysiological and molecular actions. As stated by Lydic et al., "cellular and molecular level studies of naturally occurring states of consciousness may prove to be important in understanding anesthetically induced states of consciousness" (1). This outline is intended for clinicians that are not familiar with sleep physiology and the general organization of the neural systems supporting conscious processes. More detailed descriptions will be found elsewhere.

SLEEP STAGES (2)

Sleep is not a steady state. It follows a cyclic pattern and is divided in stages that, although having behavioral and physiological specificities, are still best described by their EEG characteristics.

Stage W corresponds to the waking state and is characterized by alpha activity (eyes closed) and/or mixed frequency, low voltage EEG.

T. H. Stanley and T. D. Egan (eds.), Anesthesia for the New Millennium, 71–75.
© *1999 Kluwer Academic Publishers.*

Stage 1 is defined by a low voltage, mixed frequency EEG, with predominance of activity in the 2-7 cycles per second (cps) range. Slow eye movements are present and tonic muscle activity is lower than during wakefulness.

In Stage 2, sleep spindles are seen and are defined as bursts of at least 0.5 second in the 12-14 cps range. Spindles are generated in the thalamus and depend on the integrity of thalamocortical and reticular thalamic neurons (3). K complexes are also present in Stage 2. They have a well delineated, negative sharp wave followed by a positive component, for a total duration of more than 0.5 sec.

Stage 3 is characterized by the apparition of waves of 2 cps or slower, which have an amplitude > 75 mV. These waves must constitute between 20 and 50% of the epoch considered.

When 2 cps waves or slower constitute a value > 50%, the subject is in Stage 4. It is worth noting that sleep spindles may be present in Stage 3 and 4.

REM sleep is defined by the concomitant appearance of relatively low voltage, mixed frequency EEG activity and episodic REM. Saw-tooth waves may be present, but not spindles. The general pattern may resemble Stage 1, although physiologically, REM sleep is a special state often labeled as "paradoxical sleep" and having many features of the waking state.

CONSCIOUSNESS AND THE ACTIVATING SYSTEM   (1)

In the 1940s, Moruzzi and Magoun (4) brought into light the role of the brainstem reticular formation for the maintenance of the conscious state. This area receives collateral input from visceral, somatic and special sensory system. It sends long ascending projections through a dorsal pathway to the thalamic nuclei and a ventral pathway to the hypothalamus, subthalamus, and ventral thalamus up to the level of the basal forebrain. Various thalamic nuclei project to the cortex to form the thalamocortical system, which depends on the tonic drive from the reticular formation for its activation. Cortical projections also originate from sub-thalamic and forebrain structures and constitute another route for cortical activation.

Various neurotransmitter systems contribute to specific aspects of wakefulness. Norepinephrine and cholinergic neurons are implicated in processes of cortical activation, and dopaminergic neurons modulate behavioral activity and responsiveness. Histamine and glutamate neuronal systems as well as various peptides may be involved in the modulation of wakefulness. These systems, in turn, may influence primary processes of sensory transmission and attention, motor responses and activity, and orthosympathetic and neuroendocrine responses and regulation by which they may enhance and prolong vigilance and arousal.

SLEEP GENERATING SYSTEMS (SLOW WAVE SLEEP) (1)

Neurons of the solitary tract nucleus and of the adjacent dorsal reticular formation project into the visceral-limbic forebrain. Electrical stimulation of the caudal solitary tract induces sleep, and stimulation of various forebrain structures causes synchronization of the EEG. The thalamus is necessary for the production of cortical spindles typical of Stage 2 sleep, but not for the generation of slow wave sleep. Serotonin (Raphe nuclei) and GABA seem to be the two major neurotransmitters involved in slow wave sleep generation through widespread projections into the midbrain, forebrain and cortex.

ANESTHESIA AND SLEEP

Some recent studies tend to suggest that sleep and some anesthetic states have some underlying neuronal mechanisms in common. Here are a few examples. The release of acetylcholine in the brainstem shows some strikingly similar patterns between sleep and clinically relevant concentrations of halothane (5). Halothane also causes spindling that is not significantly different from that seen in non-REM sleep. Auditory steady-state responses sustain the same changes under sleep and anesthesia-induced unconsciousness (6-9). These evoked responses are related to endogenous gamma rhythms thought to be important in the maintenance of the conscious state. Finally, brain imaging data shows that the neuronal activity is decreased in the thalamus during sleep, propofol anesthesia and in situations of decreased vigilance (10-13). No one can conclude from these early data that sleep and anesthesia are generated by the same neuronal mechanisms, but conceptually, both processes are related in the sense that they result in a modulation of the conscious state.

Research on mechanisms of anesthesia has mostly been directed towards finding the molecular and cellular sites of action of anesthetics. Site directed research, albeit essential, is likely to offer an incomplete understanding for all the mechanisms of anesthesia. The experimental approach to sleep research has evolved towards understanding the underlying mechanistic basis of the process. It is likely that we could benefit not only from a similar approach to the problem of anesthetic action, but also from the knowledge already acquired on the neural mechanisms modulating consciousness.

BIBLIOGRAPHY

1. Lydic R, Biebuyck JF: Sleep neurobiology: relevance for mechanistic studies of anaesthesia. Brit J Anaesth 72:506-8, 1994
2. Rechtschaffen A, Kales A: A manual of standardized terminology, techniques and scoring system for sleep stages of human subjects. Los Angeles, BIS/BRI, UCLA, 1968
3. Destexhe A, Contreras D, Sejnowski TJ, Steriade M: A model of spindle rhythmicity in the isolated thalamic reticular nucleus. J Neurophysiol 72:803-18, 1994
4. Moruzzi G, Magoun HW: Brain stem reticular formation and activation of the EEG. Electroencephalog Clin Neurophysiol 1:455-73, 1949
5. Keifer JC, Baghdoyan HA, Becker L, Lydic R: Halothane decreases pontine acethylcholine release and increases EEG spindles. Neuro Report 5:577-80, 1994
6. Linden RD, Campbell KB, Hamel G, Picton TW: Human auditory steady state evoked potentials during sleep. Ear and Hearing 6:167-74, 1985
7. Plourde G, Picton TW: Human auditory steady-state response during general anesthesia. Anesth Analg 71:460-8, 1990
8. Plourde G: The effects of propofol on the 40-Hz auditory steady-state response and on the electroencephalogram in humans. Anesth Analg 82:1015-22, 1996
9. Plourde G, Villemure C, Fiset P, Bonhomme V, Backman SB: Effects of isoflurane on auditory steady state response and on unconsciousness in human volunteers. Anesthesiology In press: 1998
10. Hofle N, Paus T, Reutens D, Fiset P, Gotman J, Evans AC, Jones BE: Covariation of regional cerebral blood flow with delta and spindle activity during slow wave sleep in humans. J Neurosci 1997

75

11. Paus T, Zatorre RJ, Hofle N, Caramanos Z, Gotman J, Petrides M, Evans AC: Time-related changes in neural systems underlying attention and arousal during the performance of an auditory vigilance task. J Cognit Neurosci 9:392-408, 1997
12. Maquet P, Degueldre C, Delfiore G, Aerts J, Peters J-M, Luxen A, Franck G: Functional neuroanatomy of human slow wave sleep. J Neurosci 17:2807-12, 1997
13. Fiset P, Paus T, Daloze T, Plourde G, Hajj-Ali N, Evans A: Effect of propofol-induced anesthesia on regional cerebral blood-flow: a positron emission tomography study. Soc for Neurosci 22:357.111996 (Abstract)

AWARENESS UNDER ANESTHESIA: CURRENT UNDERSTANDING

Peter S. Sebel

INTRODUCTION

The experience of awareness during general anesthesia can be a terrifying one for the patient:

> *"The surgeon then made an incision straight down into my stomach. I just started to scream inside my head and prayed that I would not die. I could hear my skin tearing and ripping, and it felt like someone took a blowtorch to my stomach. Then the surgeon cut across my stomach. As he was cutting across my stomach, it felt as if someone took 500-pound bowling balls and dropped them right below my collarbone. I felt as if I was trapped in my brain, and screaming and praying to God and telling myself to hold on"* (1).

INCIDENCE

We do not have good data about the true incidence of the phenomenon of awareness during general anesthesia. The most recent data was obtained from a series of a thousand consecutive patients anesthetized in a British hospital and subjected, postoperatively, to a structured interview (2). There, in a non-obstetric, non-cardiac surgical setting, the incidence was found to be 0.2%. Under certain circumstances, the incidence of awareness may be higher. In major trauma cases, the incidence may be as high as 43% (3). A higher incidence of awareness has also been reported for obstetric cases and following cardiothoracic surgery, where awareness has been reported in up to 23% of cases (4).

T. H. Stanley and T. D. Egan (eds.), Anesthesia for the New Millennium, 77–84.
© 1999 *Kluwer Academic Publishers.*

CONSEQUENCES

In most cases, the experience of awareness leaves the patient with little or no adverse experiences. However, Jones (5) has suggested that 0.01% of patients who are aware suffer from pain. The consequences of this pain can be devastating for the patient. From the same patient's narrative:

> "Since my surgery, I have experienced frequent and recurrent nightmares. I often wake up in the middle of the night and see my bedroom walls turn red, or the floor turning red. I cannot go to bed without a night light on and the window blinds must be open. At times, I have great difficulty in remembering things such as finding my way to the airport, even though I made the trip many, many times. I also have extreme difficulty putting my thoughts in writing, and I forget how to spell the simplest of words. All the frustrations I have mentioned cause me a great deal of anxiety" (1).

These symptoms described above are characteristic of a post-traumatic stress disorder which may develop following a frightening or unpleasant life experience. The symptoms include anxiety, irritability, insomnia, repetitive nightmares, depression, and a preoccupation with death. Not surprisingly there may be a fear of doctors, hospitals, and particularly future operations. The patient may relive the unpleasant experience in his or her dreams. The symptoms may be severe with a prolonged course, the severity of the illness being related to the time lapse between the stressor and therapy. Many patients become extremely upset if the medical team caring for them denies or denigrates their complaints of awareness. If the patient receives early counseling, which includes an explanation of the cause of awareness, then the traumatic stress disorder may be avoided or at least be of more limited duration. It is also thought that an honest explanation and sympathetic discussion with the patient may reduce the chance of medical-legal action. The immediate involvement of a psychiatrist, psychologist, or other professional trained in the management of post-traumatic stress disorder is advisable in order to provide therapy and give practical advice. The advice may be simple, such as not to shut the patient's door or turn the lights off to avoid the possibility of feeling trapped. Treatment of the post-traumatic stress disorder may include counseling, psychotherapy, and/or psychoactive medications.

In a study of patients who were aware and referred by anesthesiologists, Moerman and colleagues found the most frequent complaints from a patient were the ability to hear what was going on in the operating room and the sensations of weakness or paralyses and inability to respond. In addition, if pain was present, its recall was unpleasant (6). Patients may particularly recall conversations or remarks which have negative connotations concerning themselves or their medical condition. The most frequently reported symptoms were those of flashbacks, daytime anxiety, dreams, and nightmares, as well as sleep disturbances.

DETECTION OF AWARENESS

In order to establish the occurrence of awareness, it is appropriate to ask a series of simple questions at the post-operative interview (2).

What was the last thing you remembered before you went to sleep?

What was the first thing you remembered when you woke up?

Can you remember anything in between these two periods?

Did you dream during your operation?

What was the worst thing about your operation?

These questions will serve to identify the occurrence of awareness in the post-operative interview. Detection of awareness intraoperatively is more difficult. It is quite apparent that hemodynamic signs are unreliable. A series of anesthetic records from patients who were aware during general anesthesia was evaluated with case-matched controls in a double-blinded manner (6).

The blinded anesthesiologists were unable to detect which patients had been aware. It is apparent that during episodes of awareness, patients may not mount a hemodynamic response and may not respond to the unpleasant episode by hypertension and tachycardia. Lacrimation and diaphoresis also may not be seen.

It is possible to detect the occurrence of awareness during general anesthesia with neuromuscular blockade using the isolated forearm technique (IFT). The technique is as follows:

After induction of anesthesia but before administration of neuromuscular blockade, a tourniquet is placed on the upper arm to above systolic blood pressure. Then, neuromuscular blockade is administered. Since the neuromuscular blockade does not extend to the isolated arm, the patient can respond to specific questions (7). This technique allows the patient to move fingers in response to command or to squeeze an investigator's fingers to command. The technique has been criticized (8) because responses may be equivocal. Responses may also interfere with surgery, and after a period of time (?20 minutes), ischemic paralysis may occur. It is possible using the IFT technique to establish EEG predictors of return of consciousness in the unstimulated paralyzed patients (9).

HOW MUCH ANESTHETIC IS ENOUGH?

We do not have good information on how much anesthetic is required to prevent episodes of awareness. For the purposes of this discussion, we will consider anesthetic concentrations in terms of MAC multiples. It is likely that patients will exhibit and move in response to surgical stimulation before they become aware. However, almost all cases of awareness during general anesthesia occur in the paralyzed patient when neuromuscular blockade has been administered. Thus, the movement response is obliterated. At an anesthetic concentration when movement is unlikely (1.3 MAC), awareness is also unlikely. Eger has suggested that perhaps 0.75 MAC is required to abolish unpleasant or fearful memories during anesthesia (10). Since 50% of patients will exhibit a movement response at 1 MAC, it seems prudent to consider anesthetic concentrations in excessive of 1 MAC as likely to prevent awareness. In unstimulated patients, consciousness appears to occur at approximately 0.45 MAC (11). However, this value is likely to be much higher in the stimulated patient.

INDIRECT MEMORY

Although this article is concerned mainly with awareness (direct memory of an event; the person experiencing the event has direct recall of it), it is also possible that indirect memory for events during anesthesia can occur. Indirect memory can be defined as a change in task performance as a result of having acquired the memory (e.g., learning) without the subject having direct recall of the stimulus. For example, if patients are played tapes of positive therapeutic suggestion during general anesthesia, they may use less post-operative analgesia (12) or leave the hospital earlier (13). These findings cannot be always replicated (14,15). It is important to note that, if patients can have indirect memory for positive therapeutic suggestions, it is likely that they can also have indirect memory for suggestions which have negative connotations. Thus, one should not make derogatory remarks about patients, the inoperability of tumors, poor outcomes, etc., during surgery. These remarks may be "heard" by the patient, processed or leading to an adverse recovery on the part of the patient. The whole issue of whether indirect memory functions during anesthesia remains controversial. However, simple steps such as described above may be taken to avoid exposing the patient to auditory input with negative connotations.

LEGAL ISSUES

Lawsuits against anesthesiologists for episodes of awareness are not uncommon. The American Society of Anesthesiologists' Closed Claim Project suggests that the incidence is 1.5% of all claims, although in other studies, the incident may be as high as 7% (16). Women were more likely to sue for awareness than men. There are circumstances under which awareness represents "a justifiable risk." Such circumstances may include obstetric, cardiothoracic, and trauma anesthesia. The occurrence of an episode of awareness is not necessarily the result of malpractice or negligence on the part of the anesthesiologist. However, where it can be demonstrated that the anesthesiologist has failed to meet the standard of care, litigation may be successfully pursued.

It is controversial as to whether the possibility of awareness should be listed in any informed consent that is obtained from the patient pre-operatively. In general, specific anesthesia consents do not usually address the issue of awareness. Informing the patient about the possibility of awareness pre-operatively does not detract from the anesthesiologist's responsibility for preventing awareness. If asked pre-operatively whether awareness may occur, it is appropriate to give an honest explanation. In high-risk patients, a pre-operative discussion of awareness is appropriate. For all general anesthetic patients, it is probably not necessary. Awareness is a relatively low-incidence phenomenon, and discussion may provoke anxiety and upset patients. However, a number of patients are already anxious about the possibility of awareness and any associated pain. In such cases a discussion may be particularly reassuring.

CAUSES AND PREVENTION

Most cases of awareness appear to be related to the use of neuromuscular blockade in conjunction with either accidental or deliberate administrations of inadequate concentration of anesthetic. During deliberate administration of low-anesthetic concentrations (e.g., when a patient is hemorrhaging severely and will not tolerate an adequate concentration of anesthetic), it is appropriate to talk to the patient and tell him what is going on. Accidental inadequate administration may be related to failure to check the machine or to monitor gas flows and agent concentrations. Infusion pumps may be inappropriately assembled or disconnected. During difficult intubations, in addition to administering increased quantities of neuromuscular blockade, additional doses of induction agents should be administered. Nitrous oxide/opioid anesthetics are probably not complete anesthetics and should be supplemented with either a volatile or intravenous agent.

Neuromuscular blockade should be avoided unless clinically indicated for surgical access. If neuromuscular blockade is used, complete relaxation should be avoided, allowing the patient to mount a movement response.

In conclusion, awareness during anesthesia is a relatively uncommon event. However, it may have devastating consequences for the patient. Conscientious administration of anesthesia with appropriate monitoring should decrease the incidence of awareness. When episodes of awareness occur, it is essential to treat the patient sympathetically and arrange for appropriate therapy as soon as possible.

BIBLIOGRAPHY

1. Tracy J, Sebel PS, Bonke B, Winograd E: Editors. Memory and Awareness in Anesthesia. Englewood Cliffs: Prentice Hall; 1993; Awareness in the Operating Room: A Patient's View. p. 349-53
2. Liu WHD, Thorp TA, Graham SG, Aitkenhead AR: Incidence of awareness with recall during general anaesthesia. Anaesth 1991;46:435-7
3. Bogetz MS, Katz JA: Recall of surgery for major trauma. Anesthesiol 1984;61:6-9
4. Goldmann L, Shah MV, Hebden MW: Memory of Cardiac Anaesthesia: Psychological sequelae in cardiac patients of intra-operative suggestion and operating room conversation. Anaesth 1987;42:596-603
5. Jones JG: Perception and memory during general anaesthesia. Br J Anaesth 1994;73:31-7
6. Moerman N, Bonke B, Oosting J. Awareness and recall during general anesthesia. Anesthesiol 1993;79:454-64
7. Tunstall ME: Detecting wakefulness during general anesthesia for Caesarean section. Br Med J 1977;1:1321
8. Breckenridge JL, Aitkenhead AR: Isolated forearm technique for detection of wakefulness during general anaesthesia. Br J Anaesth 1981;53:665P-6P
9. Flaishon R, Windsor A, Sigl J, Sebel PS: Recovery of Consciousness during General Anesthesia: EEG Bispectrum and the Isolated Forearm Technique. [In Press] Anesthesiol 1997
10. Eger II EI, Lampe GH, Wauk LZ, Whitendale P, Cahalan MK, Donegan JH: Clinical pharmacology of nitrous oxide: an argument for its continued use. Anesth Analg 1990;71:575-85
11. Chortkoff BS, Bennett HL, Eger II EI: Subanesthetic concentrations of isoflurane suppress learning as defined by the category-example task. Anesthesiol 1993;79:16-22
12. McLintock TTC, Aitken H, Downie CFA, Kenny GNC: Postoperative analgesic requirements in patients exposed to positive intraoperative suggestions. Br Med J 1990;301:788-90
13. Evans C, Richardson PH: Improved recovery and reduced postoperative stay after therapeutic suggestions during general anesthesia. Lancet 1988;ii:491-3
14. Carlsson C, Harp JR, Siesjo BK: Metabolic changes in the cerebral cortex of the rat induced by intravenous pentothalsodium. Acta Anaesth Scand 1975;57 (Suppl):7-17

15. Liu WHD, Standen PJ, Aitkenhead AR: Therapeutic suggestions during general anaesthesia in patients undergoing hysterectomy. Br J Anaesth 1994;68:277-81
16. Aitkenhead AR: The pattern of litigation against anaesthetists. Br J Anaesth 1994;73:10-21

DEPTH OF ANESTHESIA MONITORING TECHNIQUES: AN OVERVIEW

Donald R. Stanski

The word "anesthesia" was first used by the Greek philosopher Dioscorides in the first century AD to describe the narcotic effect of the plant mandragora. The word reappeared in the English language in the 1771 Encyclopedia Britannica where it was defined as a "privation of the senses" (1). After the introduction of ether anesthesia into clinical medicine by Morton in 1846, Oliver Wendell Holmes used the word to describe the new phenomenon that made surgical procedures possible.

While clinical anesthesia has been part of medicine since 1846, a clear definition of depth of anesthesia has been complex, convoluted and difficult to achieve. Plomley (2) was the first to define depth of anesthesia in 1847 using ether. He described three stages: intoxication, excitement, then the deeper level of narcosis. Later that same year, John Snow described five degrees of narcotism for ether anesthesia (3) and subsequently chloroform anesthesia (4). Snow's excellent characterization of ether and chloroform described the conjunctival reflex, regular, deep, automatic breathing, movement of the eyeballs and inhibition of the intercostal muscles. Many of these clinical signs were "rediscovered" many years later. Anesthetic practice in the early 1900s attempted to use sedative or opiate premedication to decrease the magnitude of the ether/chloroform excitement phase. Also, anesthetics with more rapid onset, like nitrous oxide and ethylene, became available.

In 1937, Guedel (5) published his classic description of the clinical signs of ether anesthesia, using physical signs involving somatic muscle tone, respiratory patterns and ocular signs to define the four stages of ether. These stages included analgesia, delirium, surgical anesthesia with 4

T. H. Stanley and T. D. Egan (eds.), Anesthesia for the New Millennium, 85–89.

planes, and finally respiratory paralysis. In 1954, Artusio (6) expanded Guedel's description of ether analgesia into three distinct planes.

Beginning in 1942, with the introduction of the muscle relaxant, d-tubocurarine, the nature of clinical anesthesia and assessment of anesthetic depth changed irreversibly. With the availability of muscle relaxants, anesthesiologists began to develop methods of controlled ventilation. They realized that the combination of controlled ventilation with moderate to large doses of muscle relaxants would allow the use of lower inspired concentrations of inhaled ether anesthesia. This reduced the risks of toxicity (cardiovascular and respiratory) and increased the speed of emergence from anesthesia, both very desirable from a clinical perspective. However, the use of muscle relaxants eliminated two very valuable types of clinical signs of depth of anesthesia, namely the rate and volume of respiration and the degree of muscle relaxation induced by the ether (7). Seven of the nine components of Guedel's classification system of anesthetic depth involved skeletal muscle activity. Thus, when muscle relaxants were used, only pupil size and lacrimation were left as clinical signs, both inadequate to judge clinical depth (8). In 1945, an unsigned editorial in *The Lancet* discussed the clinical problem of awareness that now emerged in the literature (9,10). The issue of patient awareness has remained since that time even as the types of anesthetic drugs available have changed markedly from ether anesthesia.

In 1987, Cedric Prys-Roberts (11) attempted to focus the definition of anesthetic depth onto the elements of anesthesia that were truly relevant. He first observed that depth of anesthesia is difficult to define because anesthesiologists have approached the issue in terms of the drugs available to them rather than the patient's clinical needs during surgery. Rather, he attempted to focus the definition of anesthesia depth on the body's responses to noxious stimuli, which he defines as factors that cause potential or actual cell damage, whether mechanical, chemical or thermal.

More recently, Kissin (12) expanded on the concepts presented by Prys-Roberts. He begins by indicating that a wide spectrum of pharmacological actions via different drugs can be used to create the general anesthetic state, including analgesia, anxiolysis, amnesia, unconscious and suppression of somatic motor, cardiovascular and hormonal responses to the stimulation of surgery. This spectrum of effects that constitute the state of general anesthesia should not be regarded as several components of anesthesia resulting from one anesthetic action, but represents separate pharmacological actions, even if the anesthesia is produced by one drug. Kissin believes that if one understands general anesthesia as a spectrum of separate pharmacological actions that vary according to the goals of anesthesia, then the diversity of pharmacological actions that in combination provide anesthesia makes it almost impossible to determine the potency of different actions with one measure.

Kissin and Prys-Roberts' concepts, coupled with a recent series of scientific publications to be indicated below, suggest that depth of anesthesia can only be defined by examining specific noxious stimuli and defined clinical responses under specific pharmacological conditions. With the currently available anesthetic drugs in anesthetic practice, it is necessary to use at least two anesthetic drugs, a hypnotic (inhalational e.g., isoflurane; or intravenous, e.g., propofol) and an analgesic (opiate). What is the evidence for this statement?

Although the minimum alveolar concentration concept developed by Eger and colleagues has been a powerful scientific and clinical tool to understand inhalational anesthetic clinical pharmacology, recent studies by Zbinden et al. (13,14) have changed our understanding of this anesthetic class. Zbinden et al. have shown that when isoflurane is given as the sole anesthetic and both movement and hemodynamic responses are examined for defined noxious stimuli, increasing isoflurane concentrations can prevent purposeful movement. It cannot prevent significant hemodynamic responses of hypertension and tachycardia, even at very high end-tidal concentrations of isoflurane. Glass and colleagues have shown that when opiates are added to inhalational anesthetics to obtain hemodynamic control at clinically acceptable inhalational anesthetic concentrations, marked reductions of the MAC occur (15,16). Isoflurane MAC decreases 39% at a constant fentanyl plasma concentration of 1 ng/ml and 63% at a constant fentanyl plasma concentration of 3 ng/ml.

Similar information is available for the opiates. Hug and colleagues (17,18) have demonstrated that opiates are not complete anesthetics when given alone. A second anesthetic drug (nitrous oxide, inhalational anesthetic or intravenous hypnotic) must be added to the opiate to obtain a clinically adequate state. Vuyk et al. have demonstrated a similar finding by examining the interaction of propofol and alfentanil (19,20). They have demonstrated that as plasma concentrations of propofol increase, there is a very marked decrease of the alfentanil requirement due to a synergistic interaction between propofol and the opiates.

Recent editorials (21,22) have concluded that only by quantifying the anesthetic drug interactions will further understanding and definition of anesthetic depth occur. These interactions must capture the two components of an anesthetic: the hypnotic aspect that can be created with the inhalational anesthetics or the intravenous hypnotics, and an analgesic component as generated from opiates.

What can we conclude from this review of the history of attempting to define anesthetic depth over the past one and one-half centuries? The definition of anesthesia and depth of anesthesia has been one of the most controversial, emotional and subjective aspects of the speciality of anesthesia. With ether anesthesia given with spontaneous ventilation, clinical signs of anesthetic depth were clear and awareness did not occur. With the introduction of muscle relaxants and the modern generation of inhaled and intravenous anesthetic drugs, awareness and recall became a predictable event in anesthetic care. The understanding and definition of anesthesia have evolved very slowly. Only recently have investigators recognized that depth of anesthesia can only be defined by examining specific noxious stimuli relative to defined clinical responses under specific pharmacological conditions. Clinically adequate anesthesia requires two drugs, a hypnotic and analgesic. Finally, an understanding of the interactions of the hypnotic and analgesic components of anesthetic drugs is fundamental to further understanding of anesthetic depth.

REFERENCES

1. White DC: Anesthesia, a privation of the senses. A historical introduction and some definitions. In Rosen M, Lunn JN, ed. Consciousness, Awareness and Pain in General Anesthesia. Butterworths, London, 1987
2. Plomley F: Operations upon the eye. Letter, Lancet 1:134, 1847
3. Snow J: On the inhalation of the vapors of ether in surgical operations. Containing a description of the various stages of etherization and a statement of the results of nearly eighty

operations in which ether has been employed in St. George's and the University College Hospitals. John Churchill, London, 1847

4. Snow J: On chloroform and other anesthetics. John Churchill, London, 1858

5. Guedel AE: Inhalational Anesthesia. A Fundamental Guide. Macmillan, New York, 1937

6. Artusio JF: Diethyl ether analgesia, a detailed description of the first stage of ether anesthesia in man. J Pharmacol Exp Ther 111:343, 1954

7. Robson JG: Measurement of depth of anesthesia. Br J Anaesth 41:785, 1969

8. Thomas WD, Runciman WB: Monitoring depth of anesthesia. Anaesth Intensive Care 16:69,1988

9. Editorial. Curare in anaesthesia. Lancet 2:81, 1945

10. Winterbottom EG: Insufficient anaesthesia (letter to editor). Br. Med J 1:247,1950

11. Prys-Roberts C: Anaesthesia, a practical or impossible construct? Br J Anaesth. 59:1341, 1987

12. Kissin I: General anesthetic action, an obsolete notion? Anesth Analg 76:215,1993

13. Zbinden AM, Maggiorini M, Peterson-Felix S, et al: Anesthetic depth defined using multiple noxious stimuli during isoflurane/oxygen anesthesia 1. Motor reactions. Anesthesiology 80:253, 1994

14. Zbinden AM, Petersen-Felix S, Thompson DA: Anesthetic depth defined using multiple noxious stimuli during isoflurane/oxygen anesthesia 2. Hemodynamic responses. Anesthesiology 80:261, 1994

15. Glass PSA, Gan TJ, Howell S, Ginsberg H: Drug interactions: volatile anesthetics and opiates. J Clin Anesth 9:18S, 1997

16. McEwan AI, Smith C, Dyar O, et al: Isoflurane minimum alveolar concentration reduction by fentanyl. Anesthesiology 78:864, 1993

17. Murphy MR, Hug CC Jr: The anesthetic potency of fentanyl in terms of its reduction of enflurane MAC. Anesthesiology 57:485,1982

18. Hall RI, Murphy MR, Hug CC Jr: The enflurane-sparing effect of sufentanil in dogs. Anesthesiology 67:518, 1987

19. Vuyk J, Lim T, Engbers FHM, et al: The pharmacodynamic interaction of propofol and alfentanil during lower abdominal surgery in women. Anesthesiology 83:8, 1995

20. Vuyk J, Lim T, Engbers FHM, et al: Pharmacodynamics of alfentanil as a supplement to propofol or nitrous oxide for lower abdominal surgery in female patients. Anesthesiology 78:1036,1993

21. Stanski DR, Shafer SL: Quantifying anesthetic drug interactions: implications for drug dosing. Anesthesiology 83:1, 1995

22. Glass PAS: Anesthetic drug interactions: an insight into general anesthesia, it's mechanisms and dosing strategies. Anesthesiology 88:5, 1998

BISPECTRAL INDEX MONITORING TECHNOLOGY: AN OVERVIEW

Carl E. Rosow

BIS (short for Bispectral Index) is a processed EEG parameter which has been FDA-approved as a measure of the hypnotic effects of anesthetic drugs. Several large trials show that BIS correlates well with drug-induced sedation, amnesia, and loss of consciousness.

Monitoring the central nervous system effects of anesthetic drugs has been a "holy grail" of anesthesia for decades. The anesthesia practitioner can be forgiven for some healthy skepticism about "depth of anesthesia" monitors – so many have been proposed, promoted (and discarded) without adequate supporting data. Even if such a monitor could be made, it is not clear how it would be used in the majority of cases: most anesthetics are still titrated using cardiovascular toxicity as a guide to overall effect. There is rarely any attempt to measure drug effect on the target organ.

THE MEASUREMENT OF "ANESTHESIA"

General anesthesia aims to produce *hypnosis* (sleep, lack of awareness or recall), *analgesia* (decreased autonomic or somatic response to pain), and a *quiet surgical field* (lack of movement, muscle relaxation). Unfortunately, the distinction is often blurry in the operating room: patient responses like hypertension or movement do not specifically indicate the need for analgesia versus hypnosis. Which of these things should be used as a standard against which to calibrate an anesthetic monitor?

The initial work on BIS attempted to find an EEG measure which would predict *movement*. Lack of a movement response to skin incision is the customary way to define anesthetic potency (MAC) for volatile

91

T. H. Stanley and T. D. Egan (eds.), Anesthesia for the New Millennium, 91–97.
© 1999 *Kluwer Academic Publishers.*

anesthetics, and it is also thought to predict amnesia and unconsciousness produced by these drugs. We now know that suppression of movement is largely mediated by anesthetic actions on the spinal cord; most I.V. anesthetics do not have a particularly good correlation between actions on the cord and higher brain centers. For example, thiopental and propofol can produce sleep and large changes in the cortical EEG without suppressing movement; opioids, on the other hand, may suppress movement at doses which have only small EEG effects. The research on BIS during the last four years was therefore directed at creating a measure which tracks *sedation/hypnosis* and *recall* – endpoints which are likely to be reflected in the cortical EEG.

THEORETICAL BASIS FOR BIS

Natural sleep and general anesthesia are associated with a decrease in the average EEG frequency and an increase in the average power. This information can be derived mathematically to create the so-called "power spectrum." Many attempts have been made to track anesthesia by distilling the power spectrum to a single number (median frequency, relative delta power, spectral edge frequency). For most anesthetics, these measurements are hard to use because they do not bear a simple relationship to dose. For example, low doses of benzodiazepines or propofol usually cause high frequency activation, resulting in a net increase in power spectrum frequency measures. On the other hand, large doses of thiopental or volatile agents can cause burst suppression and a net decrease in power. This means that power spectrum-derived measurements are most likely to become ambiguous when the patient is too light or too deep!

The BIS is also a single number which incorporates information on EEG power and frequency, but it includes additional information derived from a mathematical technique called bispectral analysis.

ü Bispectral analysis determines the components of the EEG which are due to harmonic and phase relationships ("bicoherence") and thus can provide more information between cortical and subcortical neural generators. Bicoherence patterns in the EEG change with increasing amounts of anesthetic drugs.

ü *BIS is an empirical, statistically derived measurement.* A large number of EEGs were obtained in subjects who had received hypnotic drugs. These were statistically analyzed to make a combination of EEG features which best predicted whether the subject was awake or asleep. The statistical model was transformed into a linear, dimensionless scale from 0 to 100 (lower number = more hypnotic effect). Finally, the scale was validated on a different group of EEGs.

ü BIS measures a state of the brain, not a concentration of a particular drug. It does not appear to be influenced by which anesthetic agent is being measured. A low value for BIS indicates hypnosis irrespective of how it was produced: BIS can be decreased during natural sleep, although not to the extent seen with high doses of anesthetic agents.

CLINICAL VALIDATION IN VOLUNTEERS

A series of volunteer trials were conducted to validate BIS. Healthy subjects were given increasing doses of propofol, midazolam, isoflurane, or the combinations midazolam-alfentanil, propofol-alfentanil, or propofol-nitrous oxide. The anesthetic agents were increased and decreased in stepwise fashion targeting specific effect site concentrations. BIS was measured continuously, and at each step drug concentrations were measured, and clinical measurements of sedation/hypnosis and memory were obtained. BIS proved to be an extraordinarily good predictor of hypnotic state and free recall, and it significantly outperformed measured or targeted blood concentrations. For all agents tested, logistic regression curves have been constructed to display the probability of response to voice and the probability of recall as a function of BIS. Overall, *a BIS value below 60 is associated with an extremely low probability of response to verbal command.* This relationship is nearly identical for all of the hypnotic agents tested, and it does not vary significantly over time or when two anesthetic drugs are combined. Free recall for word or picture cues is lost when the BIS is higher than 60, suggesting that memory impairment occurs prior to loss of consciousness.

UTILITY TRIALS IN PATIENTS

The ability of BIS to predict return of consciousness following induction of anesthesia was tested in surgical patients. After a single induction dose of propofol or thiopental, BIS was monitored continuously, and patients were assessed at intervals by asking them to squeeze the investigator's fingers twice. Although the intensity and duration of drug effect varied considerably, the return of consciousness occurred consistently when the BIS rose above 60. BIS < 65 indicated a probability < 5% that responsiveness would return within 50 sec. Changes in hemodynamics, in contrast, were poor predictors for response.

A multicenter study of 240 patients was undertaken to determine prospectively whether the addition of BIS monitoring would improve clinical outcomes. The hypothesis was that during standard practice (SP) patients are given more anesthetic than they need, in order to ensure lack of awareness. BIS monitoring should therefore reduce hypnotic drug usage and improve recovery by making titration more accurate. The design was randomized, third-party blinded; patients were given balanced alfentanil, propofol, nitrous-oxide relaxant anesthesia because it allowed independent titration of analgesia and hypnosis. Anesthesiologists were told to provide a safe anesthetic with the fastest possible recovery. In the BIS group, propofol was titrated to produce a BIS between 45 and 60, and this was raised to 60-70 during the last 15 min of the procedure. In the SP group, propofol was titrated by clinical signs, and BIS was not displayed. Alfentanil and muscle relaxants were administered as clinically indicated. The results of this large trial were striking: the use of BIS monitoring resulted in 23% less propofol usage, earlier awakening, faster time to meet PACU discharge criteria, and better global recovery scores. There was no increase in unwanted intraoperative events like hypo- or hypertension or movement.

CLINICAL USE OF BIS

The appropriate use of BIS depends upon the type of anesthetic and the clinical goals of the anesthetist.

ü *Type of anesthetic.* Titration of hypnosis with BIS is most practical in anesthetics where the three components of anesthesia are varied independently. This might be the situation during balanced anesthesia, with or without a small amount of volatile anesthetic. BIS can be used to titrate the agent producing sleep (propofol, isoflurane, etc.). Contrast this with a pure inhalation anesthetic where the agent is usually dosed to an analgesic endpoint (control of blood pressure and movement). BIS might be very low despite appropriate anesthetic "depth"; the number is still accurate, but adjusting hypnotic effect may not be desirable.

ü *Clinical goals.* For the healthy outpatient having a superficial procedure, running "close to the edge" (i.e., BIS near 60) may be appropriate. The clinician might want a bigger safety margin for major intraocular surgery, because the consequences of inadequate dosage can be disastrous. The value of BIS here is to quantify the extra effect being produced. At the other extreme, if BIS is used during Monitored Anesthesia Care, preventing oversedation (BIS > 70) may be the desired goal.

TECHNICAL POINTS

ü The BIS calculations are incorporated in a commercially available EEG monitor (Aspect Medical Systems, Model A-1050). A special electrode strip is applied to one side of the forehead to obtain a low impedance connection, and BIS is displayed on the monitor as a single value and a trend over time.

ü BIS is calculated as a moving average and incorporates 30 sec. of EEG data. This "smoothing" prevents excessive fluctuations and allows a value to be estimated when the signal is interrupted for a few seconds by electrocautery. When abrupt changes occur in hypnotic state (e.g., during induction), BIS will usually lag 5-10 seconds behind the clinical change in the patient.

ü BIS does not directly measure the effects of analgesics, although when analgesia is inadequate, painful surgical stimulation can cause cortical arousal. Since such stimulation is usually intermittent, an anesthetic which incorporates very little analgesic will often show large swings in BIS. Addition of an opioid usually reduces this variability.

ü Other things can affect BIS. Cerebral ischemia can lower BIS if it is severe enough to cause global slowing or suppression. The frontal montage used with this monitor will not detect most episodes of focal ischemia. Hypothermia (e.g., during cardiopulmonary bypass) will cause suppression and thus reduce BIS.

ü EEG contamination with large amounts of EMG will cause the BIS to read inappropriately high (a high BIS with an unresponsive patient). This can be an issue when patients are at light levels of anesthesia and receiving no muscle relaxants. EMG is displayed on the monitor to aid in interpretation of these events.

THE BOTTOM LINE: WHY MONITOR HYPNOSIS?

Obviously, all of us have gotten along without a monitor of hypnosis until now; why should we bother? The practice of anesthesia remains one of the safest and most effective in medicine. Furthermore, like all new technologies, BIS monitoring will add something to the cost of delivering anesthesia. I would argue that significant unpredictability still exists in the delivery of anesthetic care: patients still suffer intraoperative awareness (estimated at 0.2% overall, but higher in patients with trauma and those having emergency cesarean delivery), and many patients still have prolonged recovery due to relative overdosing with anesthetic agents.

In my opinion, monitoring BIS has at least **four benefits**:

1. *Improved titration of hypnotics based upon individual requirements.* The monitoring of brain effect is preferable to administering "average" doses, because it accounts for individual variability in pharmacokinetics and pharmacodynamics. In the case of expensive agents like propofol and sevoflurane, titration with BIS can result in significant savings in direct costs of drugs.

2. *Better recovery in the sense that it is more predictable.* The large clinical utility trial showed that BIS dramatically reduced the number of patients having abnormally long wake-ups from anesthesia.

3. *More rational selection of anesthetic interventions.* This monitor will help in day-to-day anesthetic decisions: "The patient is hypertensive. Should I give fentanyl or propofol?"

4. *Reduced risk of awareness.* It would require an unrealistically large database to prove that BIS monitoring reduces the total incidence of awareness with recall. The monitor has clearly been shown to predict responsiveness and recall in volunteers, and it has detected inadequate hypnosis with unexpected responsiveness in patients. Our general anesthesia patients come to us with the understanding that we will somehow provide oblivion. The availability of BIS monitoring gives us reassurance that we can actually measure that endpoint.

BIBLIOGRAPHY

1.   Gan TJ, Glass PS, Windsor A, Payne F, Rosow C, Sebel P, Manberg P, BIS Utility Study Group: Bispectral index monitoring allows faster emergence and improved recovery from propofol, alfentanil, and nitrous oxide anesthesia. Anesthesiology. 1997; 87:808-15

2.   Kearse LA Jr, Rosow C, Zaslavsky A, Connors P, Dershwitz M, Denman W: Bispectral analysis of the electroencephalogram predicts conscious processing of information during propofol sedation and hypnosis. Anesthesiology 1998; 88:25-34

3.   Rosow C, Manberg PJ: Bispectral index monitoring. In: Hines R, Bowdle TA, Eds. Annual of Anesthetic Pharmacology, Volume 2. Anesthesiology Clinics of North America. Philadelphia: W.B. Saunders, 1998:89-107

BISPECTRAL MONITORING TECHNOLOGY: CLINICAL APPLICATIONS

Peter S. Sebel

INTRODUCTION

To date, there has been no satisfactory measure of the adequacy of anesthesia. Intuitively, it is reasonable to expect that information contained in the electroencephalogram, the integrated cortical electrical activity, should contain information about the depth, or adequacy, of anesthesia. However, various processed EEG derivatives such as the power spectral edge, median frequency and other processed EEG parameters have been found not to give a clear indication of anesthetic adequacy.

The information contained in conventional EEG derivatives from the Fourier transformation contains information on power and frequency of the EEG signal. Bispectral analysis of the electroencephalogram is a non-linear expansion of the Fourier transformation and includes information on the inter-frequency phase relationships as well as conventional power and frequency derivatives (1).

IBM originally developed the technology for use in oceanographic research. It was also used by the MITRE Corporation for defense-related analysis techniques such as submarine tracking. Bispectral analysis is computationally very intensive, and it is only since the recent development of very powerful microprocessor technology that its application has been possible in anesthesia.

T. H. Stanley and T. D. Egan (eds.), Anesthesia for the New Millennium, 99–104.
© *1999 Kluwer Academic Publishers.*

BIS

Bispectral analysis of an epoch of EEG data yields a large amount of numeric data. In order to obtain the Bispectral index (BIS) the following process was utilized: Data was collected from volunteers relating EEG to clinical end-points of sedation as well as drug concentrations at steady state. The raw EEG data was reviewed and artifact rejected. Fourier analysis and Bispectral analysis were then performed on the raw EEG signal to give both Bispectral and power spectral variables. These were ranked statistically in order to provide the variables that best describe the conscious state. These variables were then subjected to a multivariate logistic regression analysis in order to weight features appropriately and develop the BIS index.

Table 1. BIS is a univariate descriptor of the EEG. It is dimensionless and is scaled from zero to 100 (see table 1).

BIS RANGE
GUIDELINES

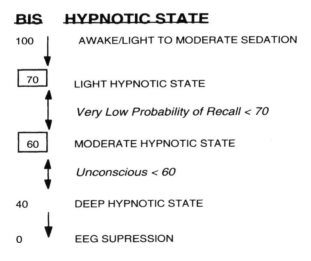

ELECTRODES

Conventional EEG electrodes are difficult to apply, and it takes a long time to achieve satisfactory impedance levels. Typically, electrode derivations have involved placing electrodes behind the hairline. In order to optimize ease of application, all BIS recordings have been derived from frontal electrodes. An electrode array (ZIP-PREP™) has been developed. These are self-prepping adhesive electrodes which result in satisfactory impedance levels with a minimum of time spent in electrode application.

MOVEMENT STUDIES

At the time of the initial studies of BIS, investigators assumed that the only unequivocal measure of inadequate anesthesia was movement in response to skin incision. Therefore, an analysis was undertaken of the ability of BIS to predict whether patients would move in response to skin incision or not (2). The first clinical study of BIS using isoflurane/oxygen anesthesia showed that patients with a higher level of BIS (65 ± 3) were more likely to move than patients with a lower level of BIS (40 ± 4). Similar data was obtained using anesthetic techniques based on isoflurane/alfentanil or propofol/alfentanil (3), and again patients with a higher level of BIS were more likely to move in response to skin incision than those with a lower level. BIS index was "tuned" to give approximately a 50% probability of movement at BIS of 50. A large multicenter study was undertaken to determine whether the ability of BIS to predict whether patients would move or not to skin incision applied across a range of anesthetic techniques and a range of institutions (4). Overall, the results were encouraging in that there was a relationship between probability of movement response and BIS value. However, there appeared to be site-specific differences. Sites in the study group that used large doses of opioids showed flatter dose responses than those which used mainly hypnotic-based anesthesia. In fact, the relationship between BIS and movement response at the time of incision when large doses of opioids utilized was unsatisfactory.

At about this time, Rampil demonstrated that MAC was not changed in rats following resection of the forebrain (5). These data suggested that movement in response to skin incision was a spinal cord reflex and that BIS, a probable measure of hypnosis, was unlikely to be able to predict this movement response.

VOLUNTEER STUDIES

It was thus apparent that movement to skin incision was not a useful indicator to use to measure the adequacy of anesthesia. Assuming that it is necessary to suppress both somatic responses and central nervous system (brain) responses, BIS was "re-tuned" to reflect the hypnotic component of anesthesia, relating degree of sedation and unconsciousness to drug concentration and EEG derivatives as described by BIS (6). This led to the current BIS index (table 1) which is independent of anesthetic agent used (with the possible exception of ketamine).

DETECTION OF AWARENESS

Data from volunteer studies suggests that at BIS of 70, there is approximately a 50% chance of awareness. These data were confirmed using the isolated forearm paradigm (7). In this technique, a tourniquet is applied to the arm to above systolic pressure before a nondepolarizing neuromuscular blocking agent is used. The patient's forearm is thus free of neuromuscular blocking agent, and the patient is able to show a motor response. Using this technique, an assessment of the point of return of consciousness (as defined by a positive response to squeeze my finger twice) was determined following propofol or thiopental. Again, at a BIS of >70, consciousness occurred. However, <70 there were no episodes of consciousness. A relationship between BIS and formation of indirect memory has also been determined. During trauma surgery, at various BIS levels, the patients were played tapes containing words. After surgery, they were asked to complete word stems. Patients completed word stems more frequently with the target words that they had heard during surgery in direct relation to the BIS level at the time of word presentation (8).

CLINICAL UTILITY

If BIS monitoring allows one to optimize the amount of anesthetic delivered to a patient, then this should result in an improved outcome from the anesthetic. That is, patients who would typically be overdosed should have a shorter recovery, and patients at the other end of the spectrum, who are typically underdosed, will receive an increased amount of anesthetic. Therefore, a prospectively randomized trial using a propofol/alfentanil/nitrous oxide anesthetic technique was undertaken to determine the utility (or otherwise) of BIS monitoring (9). Across four sites, BIS monitoring was found to result (in comparison with a control group) in 23% less propofol being used, 35-40% faster wake-up at extubation, 16% faster eligibility for PACU discharge, better PACU nursing assessments and no difference in intraoperative events. Thus, in comparison with other anesthetic monitoring modalities, BIS has been demonstrated to improve clinical outcome in terms of drug utilization and recovery.

TABLE 2. BISPECTRAL INDEX (BIS) GUIDED ANESTHETIC
MANAGEMENT

Intraoperative Response	BIS	Treatment
Increased blood pressure (BP), heart rate, autonomic or somatic response	>65	Increase hypnotic and analgesic, identify strong stimuli
Stable	>65	Rule out artifact, increase hypnotic
Hypotension or unstable	>65	Support BP, decrease analgesic, consider amnestic
Increased BP, heart rate, autonomic or somatic response	50-65	Increase analgesic, maintain hypnotic, possible paralytic, possible antihypertensive
Stable	50-65	Optimum safety and cost effectiveness
Hypotension or unstable	50-65	Support BP, decrease analgesic
Increased BP, heart rate, autonomic or somatic response	<45	Decrease hypnotic, increase analgesic, antihypertensive
Stable	<45	Decrease hypnotic, possibly decrease analgesic
Hypotension or unstable	<45	Support BP, decrease hypnotic and analgesic

In order to assess the impact of BIS monitoring on the whole operating room environment, data was collected from 490 historical controls, 345 patients during a training period, and 717 patients during a "BIS monitoring" period (10). During the training period, all anesthesia personnel were instructed in the use of the BIS and taught how to titrate anesthetics according to BIS using the BIS decision matrix (table 2).

Routine BIS monitoring was found to result in 40% faster extubation, 23% faster eligibility for PACU discharge and improved patient safety in terms of a 64% reduction in intubated PACU patients. It was found to be cost-effective (with a cost saving of $50.00 per patient) and easy to use. This study confirmed the feasibility and practicality of using BIS monitoring in a whole operating room environment.

BIBLIOGRAPHY

1. Sigl J, Chamoun N: An introduction to bispectral analysis for the electroencephalogram. J Clin Monit 1994;10:392-404
2. Sebel PS, Bowles SM, Saini V, Chamoun N: EEG bispectrum predicts movement during thiopental isoflurane anesthesia. J Clin Monit 1995;11:83-91
3. Vernon JM, Lang E, Sebel PS, Manberg PJ: Prediction of movement using bispectral EEG during propofol/alfentanil or isoflurane/ alfentanil anesthesia. Anesth Analg 1995;80:780-5
4. Sebel PS, Lang E, Rampil IJ, White PF, Cork RC, Jopling M, Smith NT, Glass PSA, Manberg PJ: A multicenter study of bispectral electroencephalogram analysis for monitoring anesthetic effect. Anesth Analg 1997;84:891-9
5. Rampil IJ, Mason P, Singh H: Anesthetic potency (MAC) is independent of forebrain structures in the rat. Anesthesiol 1993;78:707-12
6. Glass PSA, Bloom M, Kearse LA, Rosow CE, Sebel PS, Manberg PJ: Bispectral analysis measures sedation and memory effects of propofol, midazolam, isoflurane, and alfentanil in healthy volunteers. Anesthesiol 1997;86:836-47
7. Flaishon R, Windsor A, Sigl J, Sebel PS: Recovery of Consciousness after Thiopental or Propofol: Bispectral Index and the Isolated Forearm Technique. Anesthesiol 1997;86:613-9
8. Lubke GH, Kerssens C, Phaf RH, Sebel PS: Indirect memory Effects and EEG Bispectral Index in Acute Trauma Patients. Anesthesiol 1997;87:A496
9. Gan TJ, Glass PSA, Windsor A, Payne F, Rosow CE, Sebel PS, Manberg PJ, and the BIS Utility Study Group: Bispectral Index Monitoring Allows Faster Emergence and Improved Recovery from Propofol, Alfentanil, and Nitrous Oxide Anesthesia. Anesthesiol 1997;87:808-15
10. Johansen J, Sigl J: Hypnotic Titration Using Bispectral Index (BIS): Anesthetic Emergence and Recovery. [Abstract] Anesthesiol 1997;87:A434

TARGET CONTROLLED DRUG DELIVERY IN ANESTHESIOLOGY

Steven E. Kern

Target controlled drug delivery in anesthesiology is not a new concept but in fact is the clinical basis of all drug delivery in anesthetic practice. That is, the clinician determines a desired level of anesthetic necessary (the target), administers the appropriate amount of agent to achieve the desired anesthetic level (the drug delivery), and then titrates subsequent dose administration based on clinical signs used to indicate the level of anesthetic effect (the control). While this appears to be a relatively straightforward task, the complex relationships which relate the dose of drug given to the pharmacologic effect generated and the degree of ambiguity by which anesthetic level is determined create a challenge even with accurate delivery systems and rapidly acting agents.

DEFINING THE TARGET

Beginning in 1937 with Guedel, anesthesiologists have attempted to determine clinical indicators of appropriate anesthetic level, depth, or stage (1). These clinical indicators define the target against which to titrate drug delivery. This target level of anesthetic effect is produced by achieving effective concentrations of anesthetics in a patient. The concentration of anesthetic in the patient is determined by the amount of drug given and the time profile over which it is administered. These relationships are summarized in Figure 1.

The relationship between drug dose and the resulting drug concentration in the patient is governed by the pharmacokinetics of the drug being administered. In simple terms, pharmacokinetics describe "what the body does to a drug" (2). Bolus administration rapidly

T. H. Stanley and T. D. Egan (eds.), Anesthesia for the New Millennium, 105–116.
© *1999 Kluwer Academic Publishers.*

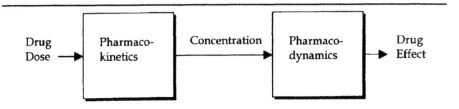

Figure 1: Representation of the dose-concentration-effect relationship for any administered drug. Pharmacokinetics and pharmacodynamics determine these relationships.

produces peaks in drug concentration in the first few minutes following the dose, followed by rapid decreases in concentration as drug is distributed and eliminated from the body. Constant rate infusions produce increasing concentrations of drug in the body which gradually approach a steady state level. However, the rate at which the steady state concentration is reached may be quite slow. For example, fentanyl concentrations are only at 20% of their eventual steady state level after a 1 hour infusion. When bolus doses and infusions are combined together, the concentration of drug can quickly increase and be sustained. The infusion rate can be adjusted to maintain a fairly constant level of drug effect. An example of this is shown in Figure 2.

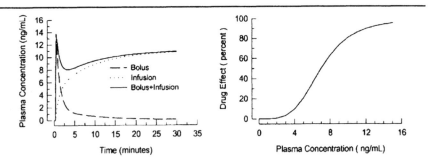

Figure 2: The pharmacokinetics of combining bolus doses with continuous infusions. The resulting plasma concentration is the sum of the individual dose curves.

Figure 3: A typical sigmoidal pharmaco-dynamic response curve. As the plasma concentration rises, the effect reaches its maximum level and plateaus.

Drug concentration is related to drug effect through pharmacodynamics, which describe "what the drug does to the body" (2). Pharmacodynamic relationships are characterized by an effect which increases with increasing concentration up to a maximum level.

This is reflected in an s-shaped or sigmoidal concentration versus effect curve as shown in Figure 3. Using the pharmacokinetic and pharmacodynamic characteristics of a particular drug, drug delivery profiles can be devised which achieve desired concentrations that produce a targeted clinical effect.

The basic principle guiding all drug delivery is that the time course of drug effect can be controlled by how you choose to give the drug. If you give repeated boluses of drug, then the plasma concentration will swing between peaks and valleys. Oscillating plasma drug concentrations will lead to oscillations in concentration at the site of drug effect. This in turn will produce oscillations in drug effect. Sometimes a rapid change in drug effect is desirable, as when a patient abruptly responds to surgical stimulation and the anesthetic effect must be quickly increased. However, in the absence of a reason to increase or decrease the depth of anesthesia, oscillating levels of drug effect are probably undesirable, with the patient being relatively over-dosed at peak effect and under-dosed at the trough. Oscillations can be reduced by giving continuous infusions of drugs rather than repeated boluses. Continuous infusions yield gradual increases or decreases in concentration. If titrated very carefully, continuous infusions will produce steady drug concentrations at the site of drug effect. This in turn can be expected to produce steady levels of drug effect.

Ideally, the target for drug delivery is some desired clinical effect. When the effect can be directly measured, such as heart rate, blood pressure, or neuromuscular relaxation, drug delivery systems can be developed that directly feedback the measured effect to an algorithm designed to adapt the drug delivery rate to maintain the desired effect. In the absence of a direct effect measurement, drug concentrations can be used as a surrogate indicator of drug effect. The clinician then must titrate concentration along the s-shaped pharmacodynamic curve until the desired clinical effect is achieved.

With inhalation anesthetic agents, this can be readily accomplished using vaporizers to deliver anesthetic agents and end tidal gas monitors to approximate the concentration of anesthetic in the subject. With intravenous agents given by infusion, this is more challenging because unlike vaporizers which control output based on concentration rather than amount, infusion pumps deliver drug based on a user set amount or rate rather than a concentration of drug to be achieved. Thus knowledge of the particular drug's pharmacokinetics is necessary to produce targeted concentrations of these agents in a subject.

HITTING THE TARGET

As shown by Eger and others (3-5), the amount of anesthetic delivered by a vaporizer set to a constant alveolar concentration decreases exponentially with time based in part on the pharmacokinetics of the inhalation anesthetic agent. To hit the desired concentration target, the anesthesiologist can simply dial in the concentration on the vaporizer. For intravenous agents, the delivery device must incorporate knowledge about the particular agent's pharmacokinetics to achieve the same kind of delivery. This is the basis for target controlled infusion (TCI) of intravenous agents.

Target controlled infusion changes the drug delivery paradigm from the representation shown in Figure 1 to that shown in Figure 4. Rather than specify a drug dose, the anesthesiologist now specifies a desired concentration of drug to achieve. The TCI device determines the temporal profile over which to administer the drug to achieve the desired concentration using a model of the drug's pharmacokinetics.

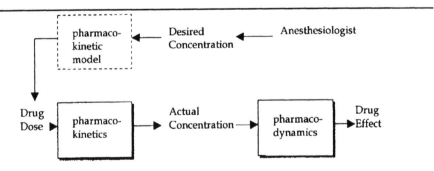

Figure 4: Representation of a target controlled infusion method for administering a drug. The system is considered open loop because no feedback is available to account for discrepancies between the desired and actual concentration.

The drug delivery profile that results from these systems is generally characterized as an exponentially declining infusion rate that drops off rapidly after an initial loading dose is administered. An example of a profile is shown in Figure 5. As one would expect, these look very similar to the anesthetic agent output profiles from a vaporizer set at a fixed inspired concentration.

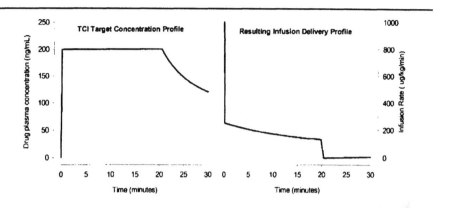

Figure 5: Example of a pharmacokinetic TCI profile and the infusion delivery profile which was needed to achieve the target concentration level in plasma.

Depending on how the pharmacokinetic model is defined in the TCI, the targeted concentration may be either in the subject's bloodstream or it may be in the biophase or theoretical site of drug effect. Many intravenous agents do not act primarily in the bloodstream but instead exhibit behavior characteristic of a distinct biophase. After an administered dose, these agents show a delay between the occurrence of the peak concentration of drug in the bloodstream and the time to peak effect achieved from that dose(6). If the TCI system is trying to achieve a desired concentration in the biophase, the drug delivery profile, while still declining exponentially, has slightly different characteristics. An example of this type of profile is shown in Figure 6. Since the biophase receives its drug from the bloodstream, the concentration of drug in the bloodstream is elevated slightly over the desired biophase concentration.

These delivery systems are considered to be open loop because no direct measure of the actual concentration is available to adapt the delivery profile so that it matches the desired concentration. The ability of the system to achieve the target level is dependent on the model accuracy.

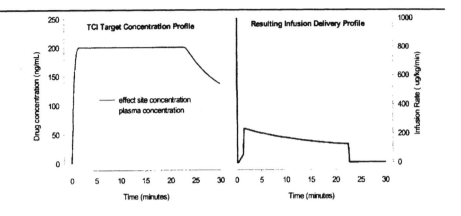

Figure 6: Example of a pharmacokinetic TCI profile and the infusion delivery profile which was needed to achieve the same target concentration level at the drug biophase or site of effect. The left panel shows both the effect site and plasma concentration levels

TCI ACCURACY

TCI systems are designed around population pharmacokinetic models for intravenous anesthetic agents. These population models are reported to have variability in parameter values that range from 10 to 50% (7). Given this degree of imprecision in the model parameters, how accurate can TCI systems be in achieving their desired concentration level?

Many research groups have developed and tested various TCI systems for delivering anesthetics, hypnotics, benzodiazepines, opioids and muscle relaxants to volunteers or surgical patients (8-12). These systems typically report median absolute performance errors, an indication of system accuracy, in the range of 20-30% (13,14). While this may seem somewhat large, it is important to remember that individual variability in response to pharmacologic agents is at least this great. As with inhalation agents, the anesthesiologist will begin with an average desired drug concentration and then titrate the concentration based on the individual patient's response. Therefore, provided that the delivery of the agent is maintained within safe limits, the absolute accuracy of these systems in producing the desired concentration is not as important as the ability of the system to maintain constant concentrations within an individual patient. An example of TCI system performance in shown in Figure 7 for the delivery of alfentanil.

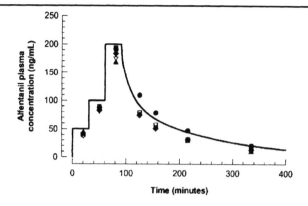

Figure 7: An example of the desired and actual concentration resulting from TCI of the opioid alfentanil using the Stanpump system. The actual concentrations shown as separate points, follow the desired profile but do not match the levels exactly.

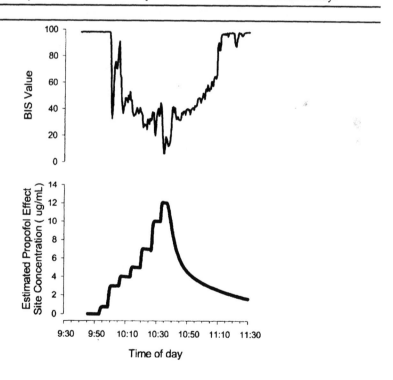

Figure 8: An increasing TCI profile for the administration of propofol and the processed EEG as reflected by the BIS monitor for a volunteer subject. With increasing propofol concentrations, the BIS value decreases in a similar stepwise fashion.

The use of TCI systems to produce relatively constant concentrations of intravenous anesthetic agents which result in relatively constant levels of anesthetic effect can be shown using the electroencephalograph (EEG). If a TCI of propofol is administered and the EEG is measured as a surrogate indicator of anesthetic effect, changes in concentration of the anesthetic produce matched changes in the EEG response as shown in Figure 8. This data was generated in a volunteer study where propofol was given by TCI in a staircase increasing profile as shown in the bottom panel of the figure (15). The EEG, measured using the Bispectral Index (16), shows a decreasing profile indicating greater anesthetic effect as the propofol concentration is increased. This exemplifies the abilities of TCI systems to step up the s-shaped pharmacodynamic curve until a desired anesthetic level is achieved.

SYSTEM CONFIGURATIONS

TCI systems have been configured by many different investigators for use in research investigations. These include the CATIA system (CATIA= Computer Aided Total Intravenous Anesthesia) (17), the TIAC system (TIAC= Titration of Intravenous Agents by Computer) (18), the CACI system (CACI= Computer Assisted Continuous Infusion) (19), and CCIP systems (CCIP= Computer Controlled Infusion Pump) (20). These research systems all have in common the use of a portable computer connected to a standardly available infusion device which is controlled via connection to the computer's serial data port. The computer contained software that included the pharmacokinetic model used to calculate the desired drug delivery rate necessary to maintain the desired drug concentration. The computer then could change the rate of the infusion pump frequently to produce the appropriate drug delivery profile. Since the use of multiple acronyms for the same basic concept is confusing, it has been recently proposed that all these systems be referred to as Target Controlled Infusion systems or TCI (21).

Two commercially available TCI systems have been developed to date and are currently under evaluation outside the United States. These are the plasma drug efflux system developed by Crankshaw and colleagues in Australia and the Diprifusor system developed in conjunction with Zeneca Pharmaceuticals in the United Kingdom (22,23). The Crankshaw system is unique in that it is designed to attain a single user-specified concentration of an intravenous agent. This limits its clinical applicability (24). The Diprifusor system is designed to exclusively deliver the intravenous anesthetic propofol. It operates as a standard TCI system with the ability for the anesthesiologist to titrate the desired concentration of propofol based on the patient's clinical response. Both these systems operate as stand-alone devices without the need for an additional computer. The pharmacokinetic model software is incorporated directly into the infusion pump electronics. It is conceivable that with the continued miniaturization of electronic components, small simple TCI systems could be available in the future.

TARGETING DRUG EFFECT WITH CLOSED LOOP SYSTEMS

Ultimately, the objective of TCI systems should be to directly control drug effect measured from the individual patients. In such systems, a generalized model can be used to initiate drug delivery which is then adapted based on differences in the measured and desired drug effect. This allows for the individualization of drug delivery to the particular patient's need. As previously mentioned, these systems have been developed for muscle relaxants to maintain a desired train-of-four response (25), for vasoactive drugs to maintain a desired blood pressure (26), and for anesthetic agents to produce a specified degree of depression of the EEG (27). These systems have typically involved the interconnection of a computer with a control system algorithm, a drug infusion pump, and a physiologic monitor for measurement of the desired drug effect. While cumbersome in their current configuration, these systems have shown that it is clinically feasible and in some cases superior to deliver drugs in this manner. With advances in sensor technology, control algorithm methods, and electronic instrumentation, these systems may offer clinical and economic advantages in anesthetic delivery in the future.

Even for delivery of agents for which a measurement of true effect is not readily available, the ability to adapt a population pharmacokinetic model based on measured concentrations of drugs in an individual patient would allow for more accurate titration with TCI systems. Maitre and Stanski have shown using simulation that the measurement of a single blood concentration of alfentanil could significantly reduce the error between the concentration of drug produced in an individual and the desired concentration predicted by the pharmacokinetic model (28). This would ultimately allow the delivery of intravenous agents with the same degree of ease and utility as inhalation agents. It remains to be seen whether the clinical and economic incentives are substantial enough to develop such systems in the future.

REFERENCES

1.   Guedel AE: Inhalational Anesthesia: A Fundamental Guide. MacMillan, New York, 1937
2.   Shafer SL, Kern SE, Stanski DR: The scientific basis of infusion techniques in anesthesia. Bard MedSystems Division, North Reading, MA, 1990
3.   Eger EI, Guadagni NP: Halothane uptake in man at constant alveolar concentration. Anesthesiology 1963; 24:299-304
4.   Mapleson WW: The rate of uptake of halothane vapor in man. Br J Anaesth 1962; 34:11-8
5.   Philip JE: Quantitative administration of inhalation anesthesia. In: Bennett PB, Watkins WD, Safety Concepts in Perioperative Monitoring. Boulder: Ohmeda 1989; pp 44-56
6.   Kern SE, Westenskow DR: Pharmacokinetic-based minibolus delivery as an alternative to continuous infusion for drugs that exhibit a biophase lag. J Pharmacokin Biopharm 1997; 25:191-208
7.   Vozeh S, Steiner C: Estimates of population pharmacokinetic parameters and performance of Bayesian feedback: a sensitivity analysis. J Pharmacokin Biopharm 1987; 15:511-28
8.   White M, Kenny GNC: Intravenous propofol anaesthesia using a computerised infusion system. Anaesthesia 1990; 45:204-9
9.   Schuttler J, Kloos S, Shwilden H, Stoeckel H: Total intravenous anaesthesia with propofol and alfentanil by computer assisted infusion. Anaesthesia 1988; 43S:2-7
10. Alvis JM, Reves JG, Govier AV, Menkhaus PG, et al: Computer-assisted continuous infusions of fentanyl during cardiac anesthesia: comparison with a manual method. Anesthesiology 1985; 63:41-9
11. Short TG, Tam YH, Tan P, Oh TE: Pharmacokinetic model-controlled infusion of midazolam: a prospective evaluation during general anaesthesia. Anaesthesia 1993; 48:187-91

12. Schwilden H, Olkkola KT: Use of a pharmacokinetic-dynamic model for automatic feedback control of atracurium. Eur J Clin Pharmacol 1991; 40:293-6

13. Varvel JR, Donoho DL, Shafer SL: Measuring the predictive performance of computer-controlled infusion pumps. J Pharmacokin Biopharm 1992; 20:63-94

14. Egan TD: Intravenous drug delivery systems: towards an intravenous "vaporizer." J Clin Anesth 1996; 8:8S-14S

15. Egan TD, Kern SE, White JL, Johnson JO: Assessing hypnotic and opioid interactions in volunteers using surrogate measures: a new study paradigm. Anesthesiology 1998; 89:A483

16. Kearse LA, Rosow C, Zaslavsky A, et al: Bispectral analysis of the electroencephalogram predicts conscious processing of information during propofol sedation and hypnosis. Anesthesiology 1998; 88:25-34

17. Schuttler J, Schwilden H, Stoeckel H: Pharmacokinetics as applied to total intravenous anaesthesia. Anaesthesia 1983; 38:53S-56S

18. Ausems ME, Stanski DR, Hug CC: An evaluation of the accuracy of pharmacokinetic data for the computer assisted infusion of alfentanil. Br J Anaesthesia 1985; 57:1217-25

19. Glass PSA, Jacobs JR, Smith LR, et al: Pharmacokinetic model-driven infusion of fentanyl: assessment of accuracy. Anesthesiology 1990;73:1082-90

20. Shafer SL, Varvel JR, Aziz N, Scott JC: Pharmacokinetics of fentanyl administered by computer-controlled infusion pump. Anesthesiology 1990; 73:1091-102

21. Glass PSA, Glen JB, Kenny GNC, et al: Nomenclature for computer-assisted infusion devices. Anesthesiology 1997; 86:1430-1

22. Crankshaw DR, Morgan DJ, Beemer GH, Karasawa F: Preprogrammed infusion of alfentanil to constant arterial plasma concentration. Anesth Analg 1993; 76:556-61

23. Engbers F, Vuyk J: Target-controlled infusion. The Medicine Group: Oxfordshire, 1996

24. Shafer SL: Constant versus optimal plasma concentrations. Anesth Analg 1993; 7:467-9

25. Kern SE, Johnson JO, Westenskow DR: Fuzzy logic for model adaptation of a pharmacokinetic-based closed loop delivery system for pancuronium. Artificial Intelligence Medicine 1997; 11:9-31

26. Westenskow DR, Meline L, Pace NL: Controlled hypotension with sodium nitroprusside: anesthesiologist versus computer. J Clin Monit 1987; 3:80-6

27. Schwilden H, Schuttler J, Stoeckel H: Closed-loop feedback control of methohexital anesthesia by quantitative EEG analysis in humans. Anesthesiology 1987; 67:341-7

28. Maitre PO, Stanski DR: Bayesian forecasting improves the prediction of intraoperative plasma concentrations of alfentanil. Anesthesiology 1988; 69:652-9

THE PRINCIPLES OF TOTAL INTRAVENOUS ANESTHESIA (TIVA)

Peter S. A. Glass

This review will provide the reader with a rational basis for the administration of intravenous anesthetics. This will be based on our increasing understanding of the pharmacological processes that provide anesthesia. The goal of any anesthetic drug is to rapidly render the patient unconscious, maintain adequate anesthesia (irrespective of any surgical intervention), and then allow a rapid recovery to the awake state. To achieve this the drug needs to provide a rapid *onset/offset* and have a *delivery system* that can readily alter the effective concentration of the drug. Over the past 30 years we have gained a greater appreciation of the pharmacokinetic principles that determine onset and offset of intravenous drugs. Classically, intravenous anesthetics have been given either as a large single dose or by multiple smaller intermittent doses for induction and maintenance of anesthesia. Recent studies indicate that intravenous anesthetics given by variable rate continuous infusions provide several advantages over intermittent bolus administration. These include: a) greater hemodynamic stability; b) fewer incidences of hemodynamic breakthrough and other signs of patient responsiveness; c) reduced need for supplemental anesthetics or vasoactive drugs; d) more rapid awakening; e) decreased incidence of requirements for naloxone or need for post-operative ventilatory support; f) decreased incidence of side effects; and g) lower total dose of drug given (1). In addition to the introduction of intravenous anesthetic drugs that meet the criteria for rapid onset/offset and are thus ideal for administration by continuous infusion, there have been technological advances that will make intravenous drug delivery as convenient as the administration of volatile anesthetics.

T. H. Stanley and T. D. Egan (eds.), Anesthesia for the New Millennium, 117–136.
© *1999 Kluwer Academic Publishers.*

When administering an intravenous anesthetic, the physician is aiming to obtain a predetermined therapeutic goal, i.e., anesthesia. The physician will administer a set dose which is expected to provide the desired response. The dose is based on the pharmacokinetics of the drug such that a therapeutic level of the agent is obtained. This set dose will provide, in any particular patient, a certain measured response, which, when compared to the anticipated response, will influence the physician as to what further dosing scheme may be necessary to provide the therapeutic goal. Thus, the therapeutic process involves the interaction of pharmacokinetics, i.e., what the body does to the drug, and the pharmacodynamics, what the drug does to the body. An understanding of each of these modalities is important in providing intravenous anesthesia.

PHARMACOKINETICS

The importance of pharmacokinetics is the ability to make use of mathematical descriptions of the disposition process to predict the resultant drug concentration within the plasma. For a two-compartment model, the plasma concentration at time T, can be calculated from the formula $CP(t) = Ae^{-at} + Be^{-bt}$. Alternatively one can make use of compartment models to calculate the plasma concentration resulting from an infusion regime. The exact solution required to calculate drug concentration using compartment models is complex. An understanding of the process involved in drug disposition, as illustrated by compartment modeling (Figure 1), does allow the clinician to provide a more rational approach to intravenous dosing regimens. The drug concentration in plasma/blood resulting from a single bolus dose of a drug administered intravenously is illustrated in figure 1.

Drug is introduced into the central compartment (blood) at a specified rate (K_{0-1}). This central compartment has a specified volume V_1. As the drug dilutes in this central compartment, it will result in a concentration dependent on the rate of drug administration/dose (K_{0-1}) and the volume of the central compartment (V_1). As drug begins to dilute within the central compartment, drug also leaves the central compartment and enters into peripheral compartment (e.g., muscle/fat) at rates specific for the drug (i.e., redistribution K_{1-2}, K_{1-3}). Obviously, drug can also return to the central compartment depending on the concentration gradients between compartments (K_{2-1}, K_{3-1}). Drug is also leaving the central compartment due to its metabolism and/or elimination (K_{1-0}). Thus, the concentration in the central compartment is the result of drug delivered into it, its volume, and drug leaving it. Volumes of distribution of both the central and peripheral compartments or rate constants into and out of the central compartment can be calculated for each drug. Utilizing these values (complex) mathematical formulae are available to predict the concentration of drug in the central compartment at time T following any drug administration regime (2).

Figure 1

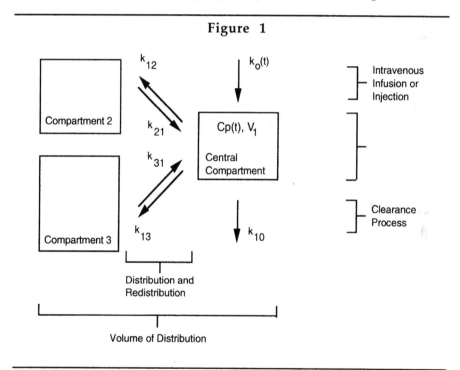

Classically texts on designing infusion schemes for intravenous anesthetics thus recommend that the initial loading dose be calculated as:

$$\text{Loading Dose} = V_1 \times Cp \qquad \text{equation 1}$$

and maintenance infusion as:

$$\text{Maintenance infusion} = Cp \times V_1 \times Cl \qquad \text{equation 2}$$

where V_1 is the initial volume of distribution and Cp is the desired plasma drug concentration and Cl is systemic clearance. This classical description of obtaining a target concentration is flawed for several reasons.

THE BIOPHASE

For intravenous anesthetics the plasma is not the site of drug effect. Even if the precise concentration for the desired effect is known, calculating the loading dose according to equation 1 would obtain the target plasma drug concentration, but the desired biophase concentration (and thus effect) would not be achieved. The site at which a drug produces its effect is termed the biophase. For a drug to reach the biophase it must distribute from the plasma/blood to the tissue of the biophase. While this is occurring, drug is also distributing into other tissues. Thus the loading dose necessary to produce the desired effect cannot be calculated using the initial volume of distribution (that includes primarily the blood volume); rather, one should use the volume into which the drug has distributed when it equilibrates with the biophase. Also the plasma concentration will not be a measure of the effect until the biophase and the plasma have equilibrated. It is possible by continuously measuring the effect of the drug and its plasma concentration to relate plasma concentration to the effect it produces in the biophase (3). When a rapid infusion of drug is administered and its plasma concentration is simultaneous measured with a measure of the drug's effect (e.g. spectral edge of the EEG or minute ventilation), it will be noted that the rapid rise in plasma concentration is not paralleled by the change in effect (3-5) (Figure 2). There is hysteresis of this relationship. It can also be noted that there is a time at which drug concentration and the measure of effect are equal (i.e., where they cross). The area under the time-concentration curve up to this point represents the volume of distribution which incorporates the biophase. This can then be measured as a percentage of the volume of distribution at steady state (Vdss) (6). The percentage of the Vdss that incorporates the biophase for several intravenous anesthetics is listed in table 1. This volume of distribution is then used in equation 1 to calculate the appropriate loading dose to achieve the desired effective concentration.

Following a bolus (or rapid infusion), if drug concentration is plotted against effect, a hysteresis loop rather than a linear relationship results. The mathematical constant that causes the hysteresis loop to collapse so that there is a linear relationship between concentration and effect is termed the k_{e0}. The constant, k_{e0}, represents the rate (time course) of equilibration of drug between the plasma and the biophase. The t1/2 k_{e0} is the time it takes for half of the equilibration to occur between the biophase and the plasma concentration. For example the t1/2 k_{e0} for fentanyl is 4.7 minutes. If the plasma concentration of fentanyl was maintained constant at 4ng/ml, then at 4.7 minutes after the infusion was initiated the observed effect would be equal to 2ng/ml. It would take four half-lives (18.8 min) before the biophase and plasma concentration are almost equal.

Figure 2

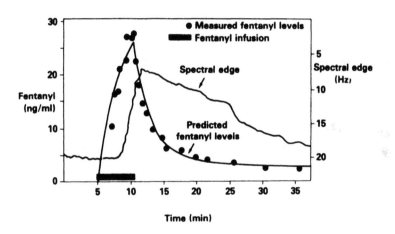

Figure 2. This figure demonstrates the simultaneous fentanyl plasma concentration and spectral edge of the electroencephalogram (a measure of drug effect). Note drug plasma concentration does not reflect effect but rather there is hysteresis of the plasma concentration to effect relationship. Figure reproduced with permission from Scott JC, Ponganis KV, Stanski DR: Quantitation of narcotic effect: the comparative pharmacodynamics of fentanyl and alfentanil. Anesthesiology 62:234-41,1985

The time to the peak effect of a drug following a bolus is also a function of the drugs' k_{e0} (and its disposition). A drug having a short t1/2 k_{e0} will have a rapid onset to peak effect. It is important for clinicians to be knowledgeable of the time to peak effect for each of the intravenous drugs. With a rapid sequence induction, for example, it is desirable to use drugs with a rapid onset like thiopental (time to peak effect-100 seconds) and alfentanil (82 seconds) so that loss of consciousness is rapid and both peak at the same time, ablating the response during laryngoscopy and endotracheal intubation. If fentanyl (time to peak effect, 216 seconds) rather than alfentanil is administered at the same time as thiopental and succinylcholine, its effect will not be maximal at the time of the greatest stimulus (intubation), and this is likely to result in initial hypertension following laryngoscopy and then hypotension as fentanyl reaches its peak effect when stimuli are minimal. In addition, when giving intravenous drugs by intermittent bolus, the interval between doses needs to be of sufficient duration so that the peak effect of the drug is observed prior to administering the next dose of the drug. For example, if 2 doses of midazolam are given 1 minute apart, i.e. prior to observing the peak effect of the drug, the plasma concentration will peak prior to the second dose but the effect has not, and thus the effect continues to rise resulting in the second dose producing greater sedation than anticipated from the first dose. A knowledge of the k_{e0} allows for the rational choice of a drug and the timing of administration of drugs used to provide anesthesia. The k_{e0} values for intravenous anesthetics are listed in table 2. *(Base loading dose on volume of distribution incorporating the biophase; base drug choice and timing on knowledge of the drug's k_{e0} value and its time to peak effect.)*

MULTI-COMPARTMENT MODELS IN DOSING STRATEGIES

The infusion scheme as formulated in equation 2 will maintain the precise plasma drug concentration if the decrease in plasma drug concentration only occurs as a result of metabolic clearance processes (i.e. the drug does not distribute from the blood/plasma to other tissues; this represents a drug whose disposition can be described using a single compartment). This is not true for any of the drugs used for anesthesia, and thus any infusion scheme must account for distribution of drug into peripheral tissues. Drugs that distribute only in the blood or plasma can be thought of as being contained in a single compartment and thus their pharmacokinetic parameters are described by a 1 compartment model. As drugs distribute into various other tissues (e.g. muscle, fat, etc.), they do so at different rates, and these tissues will contain different volumes of drug. Thus depending on how the drug is disposed of in the body, the drug's pharmacokinetic parameters can be best described by either a 2 or 3 compartment model. When designing an infusion scheme to maintain a target concentration in the plasma, the infusion scheme must not only replace drug lost from the plasma due to the terminal clearance of drug but also account for distribution into peripheral tissues. The infusion scheme to exactly maintain a target concentration has been termed the **BET** scheme (7,8). The **B** is the loading <u>b</u>olus dose as described above. E is for the infusion to replace drug removed due to its terminal <u>e</u>limination (clearance), and **T** is for an exponentially declining infusion proportional to the rate of <u>t</u>ransfer of drug to peripheral tissues. In practical terms this implies that when administering an intravenous anesthetic, one starts with a high infusion rate and decreases it with time to maintain a stable plasma concentration. A typical example of a BET scheme used in daily practice is the infusion scheme for propofol of an initial load of 2mg/kg followed by 10mg/kg/hr for 10 minutes, 8mg/kg/hr for 10 minutes and then 6mg/kg /hr thereafter to maintain propofol at 3.5 μg/ml. (*To maintain a stable target concentration, a decreasing infusion rate based on drug disposition in peripheral tissues is required.*)

Another important pharmacokinetic principle to bear in mind when administering a continuous infusion is that pharmacokinetics are based on linear models so that an infusion administered at a rate double the initial will result in a steady-state plasma concentration two times that produced by the original infusion rate. The time taken for a new infusion rate to obtain a new plasma concentration is long (and determined by the elimination half-life of the drug). During anesthesia, rapid increases in plasma concentration are required. Therefore to achieve this, *a combination of a bolus dose plus an increase in infusion rate is needed to rapidly establish a new central compartment concentration.*

The pharmacokinetic processes within a 2-3 compartment model that determine the recovery from drug effect have also recently been elucidated (6,9). The concentration of a drug in the plasma and the biophase is dependent on those processes adding drug to the body and the disposition of drug within the body. When the administration of drug to the body is terminated, the concentration of the drug in the plasma (and biophase) will decrease due to both the irreversible elimination of drug from the body and the redistribution of drug from the plasma to peripheral tissues. Conventional wisdom has been that the elimination half-life of the drug represents the measure of how rapidly recovery from drug occurs. The elimination half-life represents the terminal clearance of the drug and does not incorporate any redistribution of drug and thus clearly does not provide any quantitative measure of how long it will take for the drug to decrease by 50%. To provide an estimation of the time for recovery to occur with intravenous anesthetics, the concept of "context-sensitive half-time" has been proposed (9). It represents the time required for the plasma concentration of a drug to decrease by 50% (for an infusion designed to maintain a constant concentration) for any given duration of the infusion. The 'amount' of distribution available when the infusion is terminated is dependent on how long the drug has been administered. Thus the duration of the half-time is dependent on the length of time of the infusion (i.e., is context-sensitive to the duration of the infusion).

Figure 3

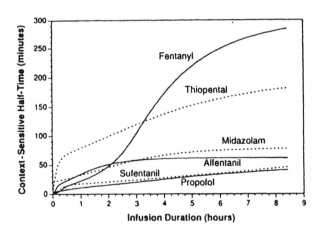

Figure 3. Computer simulations showing the time for a 50% decrease in drug plasma concentration following an infusion of varying duration designed to maintain a steady concentration. Reproduced with permission from Hughes MA, Glass PSA, Jacobs JR: Context-sensitive half-time in multi-compartment pharmacokinetic models for intravenous anesthetic drugs. Anesthesiology 76:334-41, 1992

This is well demonstrated in figure 3 which illustrates the context-sensitive half-time of the most commonly used intravenous anesthetics. In a similar vain, pharmacokinetic simulations demonstrate that the time for, a 20%, 50%, or 80% decrease in plasma drug concentration is not linear (i.e., a 20% decrease may take 5 minutes, a 50% decrease 20 minutes, and a 80% decrease 120 minutes). (Figure 4)

Figure 4

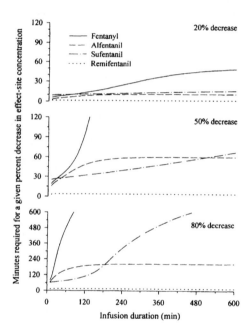

Figure 4. The 20%, 50% and 80% context sensitive decrement times for the opioids alfentanil, fentanyl, remifentanil and sufentanil. Note that the difference between a 20, 50 and 80% decrement time is very different between the different opioids.

Fortunately it appears that under many clinical circumstances a 50% decrease in plasma concentration is required from maintenance of anesthesia to the awake state and an 80-90% decrease to achieve home readiness. With this knowledge and with the use of simulations to estimate recovery times, more appropriate drug choices can be made. For example, if a 50% decrease in opiate plasma concentration following an infusion of less than 6 hours is desired, sufentanil will provide the most rapid recovery. However, if only a 20% decrease is required and an analgesic concentration needs to be maintained, then fentanyl may be a better choice.

It must also be understood that if a continuously varying plasma concentration has been administered, the context-sensitive half-time no longer will reflect the time for a 50% decrease in drug plasma concentration once the infusion is terminated. Even though the context-sensitive half-time is limited due to a narrowly defined set of circumstances (i.e., a constant concentration and a decrease of 50%), it still provides a better guide to the termination of an infusion of an intravenous anesthetic than previously estimated by the elimination half-life. (*The context-sensitive half-time rather than the elimination half-life provides a guide for both the choice of drug, with respect to the desired rate of recovery from drug effect, and an indication of when to terminate an infusion prior to the end of surgery.*)

PHARMACODYNAMICS

To assess what the drug does to the body, it is important to establish, like MAC, a measure of the concentration-effect response of the intravenous anesthetics. This measure has been termed the Cp_{50} and represents the plasma concentration (once equilibration between the plasma and biophase has occurred) that will prevent a predefined response (e.g., movement) to a given stimulus (e.g., skin incision) in 50% of patients. The Cp_{50} was first defined for alfentanil in the presence of 66% nitrous oxide for a variety of anesthetic and surgical stimuli (10) (Table 3). From these results it is evident that the required anesthetic concentration for adequate anesthesia varies markedly according to the surgical stimulus. The highest concentrations are required for endotracheal intubation. The concentration of alfentanil required for skin closure is less than that required for skin incision or spontaneous ventilation. This allows the opioid to be gradually titrated downwards towards the end of the procedure. More recently the Cp_{50} for skin incision for fentanyl (in the presence of 70% nitrous oxide) has also been defined (11) (Table 3). The IC_{50}, the steady-state plasma concentration that causes a 50% slowing of the maximal EEG has been defined for alfentanil, fentanyl, sufentanil and several newer opioids and hypnotics (4,12-17) (Table 3). The IC_{50} is not an anesthetic measure of effect, but there appears to be a strong relationship between the IC_{50} and the Cp_{50}. The IC_{50} of opioids is generally 1.5 times greater than their Cp_{50} when combined with 66% nitrous oxide. It would also appear that even though the Cp_{50} for all the various stimuli have not been defined for fentanyl or sufentanil, these can generally be estimated from those of alfentanil using an appropriate scaling factor, e.g., the Cp_{50} of alfentanil for spontaneous ventilation is approximately half of the Cp_{50} skin incision. The Cp_{50} for spontaneous ventilation of fentanyl can thus be estimated as 2.1 ng/ml, approximately half of its Cp_{50} skin incision (4.2ng/ml). The Cp_{50} for loss of consciousness and skin incision have also been defined for the hypnotics thiopental and propofol (Table 3).

Although the Cp_{50} can be defined, it is important to realize that each individual will display a different effect for a given concentration. Or stated in the reverse, for a given effect, different patients will require different concentrations of a given intravenous anesthetic. Thus it is imperative with intravenous anesthetics that they are titrated to each individual's need as well as to the surgical stimulus.

DRUG INTERACTIONS IN PROVIDING ANESTHESIA

To date there is no drug that provides all the components of anesthesia (i.e., hypnosis, analgesia, and amnesia). Thus to provide an adequate state of anesthesia, hypnotics and analgesics are generally combined. Combinations of opiate and hypnotic are used both for the induction and maintenance of anesthesia. There are now numerous excellent studies demonstrating the interaction of a variety of combinations of drugs that may be used for the induction of anesthesia. For loss of consciousness, the combination of benzodiazepine and either an opiate or another hypnotic anesthetic results in a marked synergistic interaction (i.e., the dose required of each drug when used in combination is markedly less than that predicted from the doses required of each drug for the same effect when used alone) (18-20). Opiates also tend to produce a synergistic interaction with other intravenous anesthetics for loss of consciousness, but this interaction is much less (21-26).

To characterize the interaction for the maintenance of anesthesia between opiates and anesthetics, the reduction in MAC or Cp50 (minimum concentration that is in equilibrium with the biophase that will prevent purposeful movement in 50% of patients to skin incision) has been studied (27) (see chapter on volatile opioid drug interactions). The MAC reduction of isoflurane by the opiates (fentanyl, sufentanil, alfentanil and remifentanil) is remarkably similar to the reduction in Cp50 of propofol by fentanyl or alfentanil (24,25). This interaction demonstrated a marked synergistic effect at low (analgesic) opiate concentrations and a ceiling effect at higher opiate concentrations. (See manuscript on Drug Interactions for more detailed explanation of the clinical implications of these interactions in maintaining anesthesia.)

Variability in sensitivity from patient to patient, the differing concentrations required for different stimuli, and the variable interaction between various intravenous anesthetics make it imperative that the clinician closely and continuously observe his or her patient and titrate the intravenous anesthetics to required dynamic effect.

Some typical infusion schemes for intravenous hypnotics, opiates and neuromuscular blockers are provided in Tables 4-7.

DRUG DELIVERY SYSTEMS

With the increasing interest in intravenous anesthesia, drug delivery systems that accommodate the pharmacokinetic and pharmacodynamic principles outlined above become necessary.

Realizing that it was more appropriate to administer anesthetics continuously to provide a more stable concentration, the uncalibrated vaporizer was developed. Similarly, for the intravenous drugs, administration pumps have been developed to provide a continuous infusion. Of particular note is the recent introduction of calculator pumps which are capable of making simple arithmetic calculations so that the user can enter the patient's weight and drug concentration and then administer the drug in terms of dose per unit weight or dose per unit weight per unit time. As drug effect is determined by drug concentration, it is desirable to have a delivery system that will provide an appropriate concentration at the effect site (or at least within the plasma). To this end, pharmacokinetic model-driven drug infusion devices that incorporate mathematical models to achieve a target concentration have recently been developed (28-31). These systems consist of a host computer and infusion pump and have been given numerous names according to the investigator group, e.g., CACI (Computer Assisted Continuous Infusion), TCI (Target Controlled Infusion), or CCIP (Computer Controlled Infusion Pump) (1). The first commercially available software (Diprifusor) to be incorporated into a pump for the administration of propofol has just been released in Europe (32). The host computer is linked to an infusion pump via a communication port. The host computer software provides a pharmacokinetic simulation and infusion algorithm. The anesthesiologist enters a desired target concentration by means of a keyboard or dial. The computer performs a pharmacokinetic simulation (based on the pharmacokinetic parameters of the drug and the drug dose delivered) to provide a predicted plasma concentration. The infusion rate required to obtain or maintain the target concentration over the next time period (between 3-15 seconds depending on the device) is then calculated either by an exact solution or by interpolation. This infusion rate is then communicated electronically to the infusion pump which then delivers this infusion rate to the patient. At the same time, the infusion rate actually administered by the infusion pump is communicated electronically to the pharmacokinetic simulation so that a new predicted plasma concentration can be calculated. This new predicted plasma concentration is again compared with the desired concentration and the process is then repeated every few seconds. At any point in time the anesthesiologist can alter, via the keyboard/dial, the target concentration. The system can be used to titrate up or down the desired concentration of the anesthetic, much like a vaporizer. Depending on the device, the target concentration may either be a plasma or effect site concentration. In addition, several devices will also display or allow the user to query for a context-sensitive decrement time.

The value of a pharmacokinetic model-driven infusion system are apparent in its ability to rapidly obtain a desired plasma concentration as well as to titrate the concentration according to the dynamic response. It must however be stressed that such devices provide a predicted plasma concentration which may vary from the actual measured concentration. The major source of error between the predicted/target concentration and the measured concentration when using the device is due to the difference between the patient's pharmacokinetics and the pharmacokinetic parameters utilized within the software. Several studies have evaluated the accuracy of these devices in delivering propofol, fentanyl, and alfentanil. It appears that if an optimal set of kinetic parameters are utilized, the measured concentration of approximately two-thirds of the samples will be within ± 30% of the concentration predicted by the device.

An improved understanding of pharmaco-kinetics and pharmacodynamics, the development of more suitable intravenous drug delivery systems, and the introduction of more suitable anesthetic drugs has led to intravenous anesthesia's playing a more dominant role in anesthetic practice. With increasing concern over operating room and global pollution, the use of intravenous anesthesia becomes more attractive. Although there are few comparative studies on intravenous versus inhalational anesthesia, it would appear that they are at least comparable. As familiarity with intravenous techniques is combined with newer drugs and delivery systems, advantages to intravenous anesthesia may well be realized. It is therefore important to appreciate the pharmacokinetic and pharmacodynamic principles involved in providing intravenous anesthesia and to have a knowledge of the basic dosing schemes and delivery devices required to provide an intravenous anesthetic. IC50 is the steady-state serum concentration in equilibration with the effect compartment that causes a 50% slowing of the maximal EEG. Cp50 skin incision is the steady-state plasma concentration in equilibration with the effect compartment that will prevent a somatic or autonomic response in 50% of patients. Cp50 LOC is the steady-state plasma concentration in equilibration with the effect compartment which provides absence of a response to a verbal command in 50% of patients. Cp50 Spont Vent is the steady-state plasma concentration in equilibration with the effect compartment that is associated with adequate spontaneous ventilation in 50% of patients. MEAC is the minimum effective plasma concentration providing post-operative analgesia. Values in () are estimated by scaling to the alfentanil Cp50 (see text for details).

TABLE 1. THE VOLUME OF DISTRIBUTION AT THE TIME OF PEAK EFFECT

Drug	V 1 (liters)	% of peak concentration	Vd peak effect (liters)
Fentanyl	12.7	17%	75
Alfentanil	2.19	37%	5.7
Sufentanil	17.8	20%	89
Propofol	6.7	18%	37

TABLE 2. THE $t_{1/2}$ ke0 AND TIME TO PEAK DRUG EFFECT FOLLOWING A BOLUS DOSE

Drug	Time to peak effect (min)	$t_{1/2}$ ke0 (min)
Fentanyl	3.6	4.7
Alfentanil	1.4	0.9
Sufentanil	5.6	3
Propofol	2.2	2.4
Thiopental	1.7	1.5
Midazolam	2.8	4
Etomidate	2	1.5

TABLE 3. STEADY STATE CONCENTRATIONS FOR PRE-DEFINED EFFECTS

Drug	IC50 (± SD)	Cp50 incision or painful stimulus	Cp50 LOC (± SD)	Cp50 Spont Vent (± SD)	50% Reduction in Isoflurane MAC	MEAC
Alfentanil (ng/ml)	520 ± 123	241 ± 16		226 ± 10	50	10
Fentanyl (ng/ml)	6.9 ± 1.9	4.2		(3-4)	1.67	0.7
Sufentanil (ng/ml)	0.68 ± 0.31	(0.3-0.4)		(0.3-0.4)	0.145	0.04
Remifentanil (ng/ml)	14.7	(3-6)			1.3	(0.5-1)
Thiopental (µg/ml)	17.9	39.8 ± 3.3	15.6 ± 1.1			
Propofol (µg/ml)		15.8	3.4			

TABLE 4. MANUAL INFUSION SCHEMES FOR HYPNOTICS

Drug	ANESTHESIA		SEDATION	
	Loading Dose Infusion	Maintenance Infusion	Loading Dose	Maintenance
	mg.kg^{-1}	mg.kg^{-1}.min^{-1}	mg.kg^{-1}	mg.kg^{-1}.min^{-1}
Ketamine	1500 - 2500	25 - 75	500 - 1000	10 - 20
Propofol	1000 - 2500	50 - 150	250 - 1000	10 - 50
Midazolam	50 - 150	0.25 - 1.5	25 - 100	0.25 - 1.0
Methohexital	1500 - 2500	50 - 150	250 - 1000	10 - 50

TABLE 5. MANUAL INFUSION SCHEMES FOR OPIATES

Drug	ANESTHESIA (combined with 70% N$_2$O)		ANALGESIA	
	Loading Dose	Maintenance Infusion	Loading Dose	Maintenance Infusion
	mg.kg^{-1}	mg.kg^{-1}.min^{-1}	mg.kg^{-1}	mg.kg^{-1}.min^{-1}
Alfentanil	50 - 150	0 5 - 3.0	10 - 25	0.25 1.0
Fentanyl	5 - 15	0.03 - 0.1	1 - 3	0.005 - 0.03
Sufentanil	1 - 3	0.01 - 0.05	----	----
Remifentanil		0.5 - 1	0.25 - 1 (not recommended)	0.025 - 0.2

TABLE 6. INFUSION SCHEMES FOR TIVA

HYPNOTIC	Bolus mg.kg^{-1}	Infusion mg.kg^{-1}min^{-1}	ANALGESIC	Bolus mg.kg^{-1}	Infusion mg.kg^{-1}min^{-1}
Midazolam	50 - 100	1.0 - 0.25	Alfentanil	25 - 50	2.0 - 0.5
Propofol	1000 - 2000	200 - 100	Fentanyl	3 - 6	0.08 - 0.02
			Sufentanil	0.5 - 1	0.02 - 0.002
			Remifentanil	0.5 - 1	0.25 - 1.0

TABLE 7. INFUSION SCHEME TO OBTAIN 90% NEUROMUSCULAR BLOCKADE

Drug	Loading Dose mg.kg^{-1}	Maintenance Infusion mg.kg^{-1}.min^{-1}
Succinylcholine	500 - 1000	50 - 150
Atracurium	200 - 400	4 - 6
Vecuronium	40 - 80	0.5 - 1.5
Pancuronium	70 - 100	0.25 - 0.75

134

REFERENCES

1. Glass PSA, Shafer SL, Jacobs JR, Reves JG: Intravenous drug delivery systems, Anesthesia. Edited by Miller R. New York, NY, Churchill Livingstone, 1994, pp 389-416
2. Iliadis A, Bruno R, Cano JP: Dynamical dosage regimen calculations in linear pharmacokinetics. Comp Biomed Res 21:203-20, 1988
3. Sheiner LB, Stanski DR, Vozeh S, Miller RD, Ham J: Simultaneous modeling of pharmacokinetics and pharmacodynamics: application to d-tubocurarine. Clin Pharm Ther 25:358-71, 1979
4. Scott JC, Ponganis KV, Stanski DR: EEG quantitation of narcotic effect: the comparative pharmacodynamics of fentanyl and alfentanil. Anesthesiology 62:234-41, 1985
5. Scott JC, Stanski DR: Decreased fentanyl and alfentanil dose requirements with age. A simultaneous pharmacokinetic and pharmacodynamic evaluation. J Pharm Exp Ther 240:159-66, 1987
6. Shafer SL, Varvel JR: Pharmacokinetics, pharmacodynamics, and rational opioid selection. Anesthesiology 74:53-63, 1991
7. Kruger-Thiemer E: Continuous intravenous infusion and multi-compartment accumulation. Eur J Pharmacol 4:317-24, 1968
8. Schwilden H: A general method for calculating the dosage scheme in linear pharmacokinetics. Eur J Clin Pharmacol 20:379-86, 1981
9. Hughes MA, Glass PSA, Jacobs JR: Context-sensitive half-time in multi-compartment pharmacokinetic models for intravenous anesthetic drugs. Anesthesiology 76:334-41, 1992
10. Ausems ME, Hug CC, Jr., Stanski DR, Burm AGL: Plasma concentrations of alfentanil required to supplement nitrous oxide anesthesia for general surgery. Anesthesiology 65:362-73, 1986
11. Glass PSA, Doherty M, Jacobs JR, Goodman D, Smith LR: Plasma concentration of fentanyl, with 70% nitrous oxide, to prevent movement at skin incision. Anesthesiology 78:842-7, 1993
12. Billard V, Gambus PL, Stanski DR, Shafer SL: A comparison of spectral edge, delta power, and bispectral index as EEG measures of alfentanil, propofol, and midazolam drug effect. Clin Pharmacol Ther 61:45-58, 1997
13. Egan TD, Lemmens MH, Fiset P, Stanski DR, Shafer S: Pharmacokinetic-dynamic fingerprinting in the early development of GI87084B. Clin Pharmacol Ther 53(2):209, 1993
14. Hung OR, Varvel JR, Shafer SL, Stanski DR: Thiopental pharmacodynamics II. Quantitation of clinical and electroencephalo-graphic depth of anesthesia. Anesthesiology 77:237-44, 1992
15. Schwilden H, Schüttler J, Stockel H: Closed-loop feedback control of methohexital anesthesia by quantitative EEG analysis in humans. Anesthesiology 67:341, 1987

16. Schwilden H, Stoekel H, Schuttler J: Closed-loop feedback control of propofol anaesthesia by quantitative EEG analysis in humans. Br J Anaesth 62:290-6, 1989

17. Scott JC, Cooke JE, Stanski DR: Electroencephalographic quantitation of opioid effect: comparative pharmacodynamics of fentanyl and sufentanil. Anesthesiology 74:34, 1991

18. Kissin I, Brown PT, Bradley EL, Robinson CA, Cassady JL: Diazepam-morphine hypnotic synergism in rats. Anesthesiology 70:689-94, 1989

19. Kissin I, Vinik HR, Castillo R, Bradley EL: Alfentanil potentiates midazolam induced unconsciousness in sub analgesic doses. Anesth Analg 71:65-9, 1990

20. Kissin I, Brown PT, Bradley EL: Sedative and hypnotic midazolam-morphine interactions in rats. Anesth Analg 71:137-43, 1990

21. Kissin I, Mason JO, Bradley EL: Morphine and fentanyl hypnotic interactions with thiopental. Anesthesiology 67:331-5, 1987

22. Vinik HR, Bradley EL, Kissin I: Alfentanil does not potentiate hypnotic effect of propofol (abstract). Anesth Analg 72:S308, 1991

23. Vinik HR, Bradley Jr EL, Kissin I: Triple anesthetic combination: propofol-midazolam-alfentanil. Anesth Analg 78:354-8, 1994

24. Smith C, McEwan AI, Jhaveri R, Wilkinson M, Goodman D, Smith LR, Canada AT, Glass PSA: The interaction of fentanyl on the C_{p50} of propofol for loss of consciousness and skin incision. Anesthesiology 81: 820-8, 1994

25. Vuyk J, Lim T, Engbers FHM, Burm AGL, Vletter AA, Bovill JG: The pharmacodynamic interaction of propofol and alfentanil during lower abdominal surgery in female patients. Anesthesiology 83:8-22, 1995

26. Telford RJ, Glass PSA, Goodman D, Jacobs JR: Fentanyl does not alter the "sleep" plasma concentration of thiopental. Anesth Analg 75: 523-9, 1992

27. Glass PSA, Gan TJ, Howell S, Ginsberg B: Drug interactions: Volatile anesthetics and opioids. J Clin Anesth 9:18s-22s, 1997

28. Shafer SL, Gregg K: Algorithms to rapidly achieve and maintain stable drug concentrations at the site of drug effect with a computer controlled infusion pump. J Pharmacokinet Biopharm 20:147-69, 1992

29. Jacobs JR, Williams EA: Algorithm to control "effect compartment" drug concentrations in pharmacokinetic model-driven drug delivery. IEEE Trans Biomed Eng 40((10)): 993-9, 1993

30. Jacobs JR: Algorithm for optimal linear model-based control with application to pharmacokinetic model-driven drug delivery. IEEE Trans Biomed Eng 37:107-9, 1990

31. Schwilden H, Schuttler J, Stoekel H: Pharmacokinetics as applied to total intravenous anaesthesia: theoretical considerations. Anaesthesia 38((suppl)):51-2, 1983

32. Servin FS: TCI compared with manually controlled infusion of propofol: a multi-center study. Anaesthesia 53(Supplement 1):82-6, 1998

TRANSMUCOSAL AND OTHER NEW DRUG DELIVERY TECHNOLOGIES

Theodore H. Stanley

INTRODUCTION

Anesthesiologists, more than any other physicians, rely on a variety of techniques to administer pharmacologic compounds to care for their patients. More traditional drug delivery methods, such as intramuscular, intravenous, oral and rectal drug administration, while useful in most patients, may not be as suitable in others. Certainly, non-invasive drug delivery systems have several other potential advantages over traditional techniques of drug administration. When compared with orally administered drugs, transdermal and transmucosal administration systems bypass hepatic first-pass metabolism and avoid gastrointestinal degradation. Long-term transdermal or iontophoresis drug delivery systems reduce the variability of serum drug concentration profiles, eliminate peak and trough concentrations and allow for improved drug safety by reducing high plasma concentrations which often occur with intramuscular or intravenous drug administration. The latter reduces dosing frequency and simplifies dosing schedules. In addition, patient compliance is improved by decreasing the pain involved with drug delivery. Finally, some non-invasive drug delivery systems allow for "titration to effect" and thus enable rapid onset and cessation of drug administration. In this report we discuss current and future delivery systems being studied and developed for sedative/hypnotic, amnestic, anti-emetic, anesthetic and analgesic drug administration.

T. H. Stanley and T. D. Egan (eds.), Anesthesia for the New Millennium, 137–151.

TRANSDERMAL DRUG DELIVERY

The transdermal application of medications is not new in that mankind has been applying dermal ointments and creams for primarily local effects for centuries. However, the stratum corneum, 15-20 cells thick and covering over 99% of the body surface area, has proved difficult to penetrate, and systemic delivery of drugs using this route has been limited in spite of extensive investigation. Currently, there are less than a dozen marketed transdermal drugs available in the United States. A few of these include: scopolamine for motion sickness; nitroglycerin for angina; clonidine for hypertension; estradiol for estrogen replacement during menopause; and fentanyl for pain. Fentanyl has been incorporated into a transdermal delivery system and has undergone extensive evaluation for its use in the management of pain (TTS-fentanyl, Alza Corp., Palo Alto, CA).

TTS-fentanyl is designed to deliver fentanyl at a constant rate of 25, 50, 75, or 100 μg/hr. Holley and van Steennis evaluated the serum concentrations of fentanyl achieved with either intravenous infusions or TTS-fentanyl in patients undergoing major surgery. They reported that the TTS-fentanyl system provided steady-state plasma concentrations similar to those resulting from constant rate IV infusions. However, after TTS-fentanyl, plasma concentrations of fentanyl increased slowly (15 hr to plateau) and decreased slowly after removal of the patch with an apparent half-life of 21 hours.

Caplan and associates reported on their prospective, randomized, placebo-controlled, double-blind evaluation of a transdermal system designed to deliver fentanyl citrate at a rate of 75 μg/hr in 42 patients undergoing major shoulder surgery. Patients in the active group required significantly less supplemental morphine than the placebo group during the 24-hour period that the systems were in place (0.8 mg/hr vs 1.3 mg/hr) and for the first 12 hours after transdermal fentanyl removal (0.3 mg/hr vs 0.5 mg/hr). In addition, visual analog scores for pain were lower in the active group than the control group during the 24-hour period that the systems were in place and for the first 12 hours after transdermal fentanyl removal. However, the incidence of vomiting was greater in the active than the placebo groups (73% vs 30%).

In summary, transdermal fentanyl appears to reliably administer fentanyl in controlled amounts over long periods of time. However, there is a delay to steady state (15 hr) and, once the patch is removed the effective half-life of fentanyl appears to be in the range of 21 hours, probably reflecting continued absorption from a skin depot. Although residual dermal fentanyl may be advantageous for sustained analgesia, it could be problematic if drug delivery had to be discontinued secondary to over-dosage or for the treatment of drug-induced side effects. While most of the studies to date with transdermal fentanyl have been accomplished in patients experiencing postoperative pain, it is not approved for use in opioid-naive patients because of a high incidence of clinically significant respiratory depression in this population after surgery. Transdermal fentanyl is having its greatest impact on the management of long-term pain, such as that seen in patients with cancer who are tolerant to opioids. It is FDA-approved in this population of patients.

IONTOPHORESIS

Because of difficulties in the passive delivery of drugs through the skin, physical and chemical methods of enhancing transdermal drug delivery are being investigated. Iontophoresis is a method of transdermal administration of ionizable drugs in which the electrically charged components are propelled through the skin by an external electric field. Since this technique was first conceived in 1740, drug delivery from the positive electrode has been limited by the generation of H^+ ions. The H^+ ions compete for charge transport and thus decrease the amount of drug which can be delivered. In addition, the generation of H^+ ions leads to a decreased pH within the electrode which can lead to significant skin burns. Finally, the current passing from a metal electrode frequently causes its dissolution, resulting in additional competing ions within the drug delivery compartment. Because of these problems, drug delivery times are usually limited to 15-30 minutes, depending upon the current intensity and the specific drug.

Recent research leading to the development of a silver electrode and chloride solutions of different positively charged drugs have made it feasible to deliver drugs iontophoretically for 3 hours or longer. The utilization of the silver electrode allows for iontophoresis of positively charged morphine molecules while generating insoluble AgCl at lower voltages than those required for electrolysis of water. As a result, ionic competition does not occur. This advance allows iontophoresis to continue for hours without risk of skin burns or decreasing drug delivery rates.

Iontophoresis of lidocaine for analgesia for superficial surgical procedures has been reported by a number of authors. In addition, iontophoresis has been utilized to deliver corticosteroids for the treatment of painful joints. However, documentation of the use of iontophoresis for these purposes is still limited, and iontophoresis has not met with widespread use, in spite of the availability of low-cost iontophoresis units and improved electrode technology. Perhaps this is due in part to the time necessary to achieve analgesia (10-15 minutes with lidocaine) and the slight risk of burns with this technology.

Iontophoresis of morphine HCl for the management of moderate to severe postoperative pain has been recently reported. No studies to date have been reported on the bioavailability of morphine administered via iontophoresis or that of other potent opioids. In addition, no data are currently available evaluating the use of iontophoresis to deliver opioids for periods of time greater than six hours. However, this technology shows promise as a method of delivering systemic doses of potent opioids and possesses the advantage of changing the dose of drug delivered by adjusting delivery current. In addition, iontophoresis should allow for discontinuation of drug delivery with discontinuation of delivery current, avoiding the "depot" effect currently seen with transdermal fentanyl.

INTRANASAL TRANSMUCOSAL DRUG DELIVERY

Intranasal transmucosal drug delivery is another drug delivery alternative which has the potential advantages of non-invasive delivery of drugs that presently undergo extensive inactivation in the gastrointestinal tract following oral administration. The surface area of the nasal cavity in an adult is approximately 180 cm^2 and has a large blood supply, about 40 ml/min/100 gm of tissue, allowing for potentially easy access for systemic delivery of medications. To date, only a few drug preparations intended for systemic delivery via the intranasal route are available in the United States. These include desmopressin (DDAVP), lypressin (Diapid), oxytocin (Syntocinon), and butorphanol (Stadol). However, extensive research into intranasal delivery of a variety of drugs is currently being conducted.

The nasal administration of sufentanil as a preanesthetic medication has been studied in children and adults. Henderson and associates evaluated the use of intranasal sufentanil (1.5, 3.0 or 4.5 µg/kg) or saline placebo in 80 children, ages 6 months to 7 years, scheduled for elective surgery. They found that children given sufentanil were more likely to separate willingly from their parents and be judged as calm at or before 10 minutes following drug delivery than children receiving the placebo. In addition, the children moved or coughed less during tracheal intubation, required less halothane, cried less and were given fewer analgesics following surgery. However, 61% of all the children in the study cried during intranasal drug administration and the incidence of vomiting in the recovery room and during the first postoperative day was higher in the intranasal sufentanil group. In adult patients, intranasal sufentanil (10 and 20 µg) was found to provide effective, rapid sedation (onset: 10 minutes) and minimal side effects. Intranasal midazolam and ketamine have also been studied and are not uncommonly used for premedication in children before induction of general anesthesia.

Multiple factors have been noted to affect the delivery of intranasally administered drugs, including: the surface temperature of the nasal mucosa; airway resistance; atmospheric conditions; drug factors (pH lipid solubility, molecular weight, pKa); and the technique of drug administration (droplet size, site of deposition, etc.). Little information on the effects of intranasal delivery of opioids for the principal purpose of providing analgesia (such as pain following surgery) or on the effects of long-term intranasal opioid delivery has been reported; therefore, the role of this drug delivery route for analgesia remains unclear.

ORAL TRANSMUCOSAL DRUG DELIVERY

Potential advantages of oral transmucosal opioid delivery include less hepatic first-pass metabolism and improved patient comfort, convenience and compliance. In addition, since the oral cavity is rich in blood vessels and lymphatics, drug absorption is fast and onset of action rapid, when compared with oral (GI) and transdermal routes. Rapid onset of action enables titration of drug dosage to specific endpoints of effect. The mouth has three areas for potential transmucosal delivery: beneath the tongue (sublingual), between the gum of the upper molars and the cheek (buccal), and between the gum of the incisors and the upper lip (gingival). Drug permeability appears to be highest in the sublingual area and lowest at the gingival site.

Buccal administration of morphine has been evaluated and produced mixed results. In one study, Bell and associates reported on a prospective, double-blind, placebo-controlled study of buccal and intramuscular morphine in 40 patients undergoing elective orthopedic operations. Patients received either intramuscular or a buccal tablet of morphine, 13.3 mg. The tablet was placed between the upper lip and the gum above the incisor teeth and allowed to slowly dissolve over 6 hours. They reported that IM and buccal morphine provided similar analgesia following surgery. In addition, plasma morphine concentrations were similar, with the peak level being slightly higher following IM administration, but the bioavailability of buccal morphine was 40-50% greater than IM morphine. However, several reports have failed to reproduce these findings. Fisher and associates reported a wide variability of systemic morphine delivery and a bioavailability of about 13% after buccal morphine, much lower than that of oral morphine. In another double-blind study comparing IM with buccal morphine as a preoperative medication in orthopedic patients, IM morphine was more effective and had fewer adverse side effects. Certainly, morphine's relatively low lipid solubility makes it an unlikely candidate for effective transmucosal absorption. In fact, while sublingual administration of morphine provides good analgesia and a low incidence of side effects, bioavailability is poor when compared with sublingual administration of other more lipid soluble opioids.

Investigations into the oral transmucosal delivery of fentanyl have been ongoing for the past decade. Fentanyl has been incorporated into a sucrose-based lozenge on a stick (Oral Transmucosal Fentanyl Citrate, OTFC, Anesta Corp., Salt Lake City, Utah) for transmucosal delivery.

OTFC, also called a fentanyl oralet, has been evaluated as a premedicant and as an analgesic in the emergency department, following surgery, and for breakthrough cancer pain. Fentanyl oralet was approved by the FDA for use as a premedicant in children and adults before anesthesia and painful procedures. Initial studies with fentanyl oralet in adult volunteers and children have shown the device produces reliable sedation and anxiolysis when used as a premedication. In children, OTFC leads to rapid sedation and decreased anxiety within 30 min of beginning administration. Compared with children receiving nasal sufentanil, 61% of whom cried with drug administration, children readily accepted oralet. In addition, patients who receive oralet required less potent inhalational anesthesia during operation and less pain medication in the recovery room. Recovery times were not prolonged, but oralet administration did delay discharge from the hospital by 30-40 min in outpatients when compared with placebo controls in one study. Chief side effects of fentanyl oralet when used for premedication are postoperative nausea and vomiting. However, the incidence of these problems appears to be no greater than when fentanyl is given intravenously.

In the emergency department, fentanyl oralet provided good analgesia for patients following painful injury or illness, without an increase in the incidence of opioid-related adverse effects. Fentanyl oralet also provided effective post-operative analgesia for patients undergoing joint replacement surgery. During use as an analgesic for the treatment of breakthrough and incident cancer pain, fentanyl oralet appeared to be well-suited for this indication; the route of administration was well accepted, the onset of analgesia was rapid (5-15 min), and patients appeared to be able to titrate the drug to effect. The use of fentanyl oralet for post-operative and chronic cancer pain continues to be extensively studied. It has not yet been submitted to the FDA for approval.

The bioavailability of fentanyl oralet has been established in a volunteer study comparing IV fentanyl, an oral solution, and oralet. Peak plasma concentrations of fentanyl after oralet were twice those of oral administration and occurred earlier (T_{max} for oralet = 23 min vs 90 for oral). The overall bioavailability of OTFC (52%) exceeded that of oral fentanyl (32%). Etomidate has also been studied using the oralet oral transmucosal delivery concept. Onset of sedation is fast (5-10 min), peak sedative effects are dose-related, and full recovery is rapid (less than 60 min after beginning administration). In addition, side effects such as pain on injection, myoclonia, and nausea and vomiting are low or non-existent. Oral transmucosal etomidate is about to begin clinical trials.

FUTURE CONCEPTS

Future approaches and increased understanding of central nervous system receptors and the natural and synthetic neurotransmitters (drugs) that act or interact at these sites have enabled numerous researchers to consider ways in which more specific drugs could be developed or drugs could be made more selective. This has introduced the expression 'drug focusing.' Drug focusing addresses the concept of limitation of drug action to specific receptor sites within certain organs or specific tissues or cells within these organs. The development of liposomes, microscopic lipid bags or envelopes that could encase drugs, now provides a mechanism by which these compounds could be carried in an inactive form after injection into the blood stream. The idea of exploiting liposomes as biodegradable, slow-release packaging material for drugs was manifest in early 1969. Advantages of liposomes as useful vehicles for the purpose of delivering drugs include their biodegradability and similarity to natural membranes, and the possibility of modifying them to suit a variety of compounds and situations. Disadvantages up until recently have included the fact that liposomes are recognized as foreign and quickly dispatched to the reticulo-endothelial tissues for destruction and the ability to ensure that these lipid bags would discharge their contents at exactly when and precisely where they were desired. The disadvantages now appear to be solvable using recent developments in wave technology, computer-directed imaging techniques and photomedicine.

WAVE TECHNOLOGY, COMPUTER-DIRECTED IMAGING, PHOTOMEDICINE AND ANESTHESIOLOGY

Practical applications of the beginnings of high-tech medicine in the areas of new wave techniques, computer-directed imaging and photomedicine abound in hospitals throughout the world and in changes occurring in every day life. In medicine these developments are still largely diagnostic (nuclear magnetic imaging) but are beginning to become therapeutic (lasers and monoclonal antibodies). The question is how are or will these developments affect or alter the principles and practice of anesthesiology? The answer is by helping the specialty improve drug focusing and perhaps entirely substitute for the analgesics, sedatives, hypnotics and anesthetics we now use.

It is now clearly possible to encapsulate any of our currently available anesthetics in lipid bags. It is also possible to selectively break these lipid bags by focusing microwave, ultra-sonic or other waves on these bags so that the temperature of the membrane of the bag is only slightly increased (perhaps 1.5-2.0 °C), a temperature that will rupture the bag (Hills B, personal communication). Only the bags within the focal spectrum of the wave being utilized will break, thus the contained drugs will only be released in the desired local area. It would seem possible that laser energy could also be used to selectively destroy lipid bags (liposomes) and focus anesthetic compounds, but to my knowledge this has not been accomplished. It would also seem possible that the wave (energy) force utilized to selectively release compounds from their inactive envelopes could be focused on very precise organelles and perhaps receptor sites within the spinal cord or brain, principles similar to those evolving with monoclonal antibodies. Unfortunately, it does not appear that this is yet possible in 1995 but my suspicion is that it will be in the not too distant future.

Can the revolutionary developments in imaging technology be utilized to focus drugs or lipid bags containing pharmacologically active compounds on precise organelles in the central nervous system? The experts (Ailion D, personal communication), say it might be possible to identify the receptors or chemical components of the receptors via a technique called high resolution focusing in a few years. However, direct steering of the drug to the identified receptor seems extremely difficult. The reason seems to be related to the fact that current computer directed imaging technologies don't steer but rather orient molecules (nuclei, etc.). Having identified the location of where the drug is to act, having a mechanism to activate the drug only leaves the problem of focusing the drug on the receptor. One wonders if this final problem might be solved by attempting to design the drug to be attracted to the receptor via an antigen-antibody or similar mechanism or flooding an inactive drug systemically which is only activated by an energy source (laser) focused on the receptor.

DRUG ACTIVITY WITHOUT THE DRUG

Concepts related to affecting and particularly slowing or quieting CNS activity without use of pharmacologic compounds are not new. Indeed, it is possible to trace the use of electrical currents for the precise purpose of producing anesthesia to the turn of this century, and some authors have even traced ideas back to biblical times. More recently, acupuncture and methods of producing analgesia via transcutaneous electrical stimulation have become popular and apparently are, at least in some patients, effective. The recognition of transmitter-receptor interactions as a cause of many natural cerebral activities, the evolution of specific CNS-acting drugs which depress the spinal cord and/or brain via interference or effects on neurotransmitters, receptors or both, and the realization that drug and neurotransmitter action at receptor sites can be electrically provoked raises the possibility of producing drug action on the CNS (perhaps profound drug action) without need for the drug. Indeed, the ability to identify the receptor in vivo (perhaps non-invasively utilizing computer-controlled imaging technology) suggests that it should be possible to directly affect (depress, activate, interfere with) receptor activity via focused energy sources (on the receptor). The trick now is to identify the precise (best) energy source and set of characteristics and focus that source precisely on that part of the cell membrane to depolarize, hyperpolarize or whatever to prevent nerve conduction. Either one or both could be the desired effect. The power of current imaging technology and the ever expanding knowledge base of energy and wave sources is critical to future drug focusing. However, it is already quite clear that externally applied electrical fields can induce and/or alter depolarization in pyramidal and other neural elements. What is not clear is the range of fields that produce reversible neurological effects and the possible magnitude of induced changes. Our laboratory is currently investigating the effects of a variety of photo, magnetic and micro energy wave forms on nerve conduction. Early progress is extremely encouraging, and we now believe that anesthesiology in the 21st century will undoubtedly offer the possibility of analgesia, sedation, hypnosis and complete anesthesia without a foreign compound via computer-focused physical activation of receptor sites and/or neurotransmitter modulation with non-invasive external wave forms or energy sources.

REFERENCES

1.   Duthie DJR, Rowbotham DJ, Wyld R, et al: Plasma fentanyl concentrations during transdermal delivery of fentanyl to surgical patients. Br J Anaesth 60:614-8, 1988
2.   Gourlay GK, Kowalski SR, Plummer JL, et al: The transdermal administration of fentanyl in the treatment of postoperative pain: pharmacokinetics and pharmacodynamic effects. Pain 37:193-202, 1989
3.   Holley FO, van Steennis C: Transdermal administration of fentanyl for postoperative analgesia (abstract). Anesthesiology 65:A548, 1986
4.   Streisand JB, Stanley TH: Opioids: new techniques in routes of administration. Current Opinion in Anaesthesiology 2:456-62, 1989
5.   Caplan RA, Matsen III FA, Ready LB, et al: Transdermal fentanyl for postoperative pain management. JAMA 261:1036-9, 1989
6.   Gourlay GK, Kowalski SR, Plummer JL, et al: The efficacy of transdermal fentanyl in the treatment of postoperative pain: a double-blind comparison of fentanyl and placebo systems. Pain 40:21-7, 1990
7.   Rolf D: Chemical and physical methods of enhancing transdermal drug delivery. Pharm Tech 130-40, 1988
8.   Delacerda FG: A comparative study of three methods of treatment for shoulder girdle myofascial syndrome. J Orthopaedic and Sports Physic Ther 4:51-4, 1982
9.   Harris PR: Iontophoresis: clinical research in musculoskeletal inflammatory conditions. J Orthopaedic and Sports Physic Ther 4:103-8, 1982
10. Glass JM, Stephen RL, Jacobson SC: The quantity and distribution of radio labeled dexamethasone delivered to tissue by iontophoresis. Int J Derm 19:519-35, 1980
11. Petelenz T, Petelenz AI, Iwinski TJ, et al: Mini set for iontophoresis for topical analgesia before injection. Int J Clin Pharmacol Ther Toxicol 22:152-5, 1984
12. Bezzant JL, Pentelenz TJ, Jacobson SC: Painless cauterization of spider veins using iontophoretic local anesthesia. J Am Acad Derm 19:869-75, 1988
13. Ashburn MA, Stephen RL, Petelenz TJ, et al: Controlled iontophoretic delivery of morphine HCl for post-operative pain relief (abstract). Anesthesiology 69: 348, 1988
14. Weinberg AL, Freestone DS: The administration of drugs and vaccines by the intranasal route. Br J Clin Phar 3:827-30, 1976

15. Henderson JM, Brodsky DA, Fisher DM, et al: Pre-induction of anesthesia in pediatric patients with nasally administered sufentanil. Anesthesiology 68:671-5, 1988

16. Leigh J, Pandit UA, Rosen D, et al: Intranasal midazolam premedication in pre-school children does not cause respiratory depression or delay recovery. Proceedings of 9th World Congress of Anaesthesiologists (abstracts) II:A0823, 1988

17. Russell LJ, Aldrete JA: Intranasal ketamine: preliminary pharmacokinetics. Proceedings of 9th World Congress of Anaesthesiologists II:A0864, 1988

18. Squire: Br Med Bull 31:169-75, 1975

19. Bell MD, Murray GR, Mishra P, et al: Buccal morphine-a new route for analgesia? Lancet 1:71-3, 1985

20. Fisher AP, Fung C, Hanna M: Absorption of buccal morphine. Anaesthesia 43:552-3, 1988

21. Fisher AP, Vine P, Whitlock J: Buccal morphine premedication. Anaesthesia 41:1104-11, 1986

22. Hirsh JD: Sublingual morphine sulfate in chronic pain management. Clinical Pharmacy 3:585-6, 1984

23. Weinberg DS, Inturrisi CE, Reidenberg B, et al: Sublingual absorption of selected opioid analgesics. Clin Pharmacol Ther, Sept 1988:1988

24. Edge WG, Cooper GM, Morgan M: Analgesic effects of sublingual buprenorphine. Anaesthesia 34:463-7, 1979

25. Bullingham RES, McQuay HJ, Porter EJB, et al: Sublingual buprenorphine used postoperatively: ten hour plasma drug concentration analysis. Br J Clin Pharmacol 13:665-73, 1982

26. Streisand JB, Ashburn MA, LeMaire L, et al: Bioavailability and absorption or oral transmucosal fentanyl citrate. Anesthesiology 71:A230, 1989

27. Ashburn MA, Streisand JB, Tarver SD, et al: Oral transmucosal fentanyl citrate for premedication in paediatric outpatients. Can J Anaesth 37:856-866, 1990

28. Nelson PS, Streisand JB, Mulder SM, et al: Comparison of oral transmucosal fentanyl citrate and an oral solution of meperidine, diazepam, and atropine for premedication in children. Anesthesiology 70: 616-21, 1989

29. Stanley TH, Hague B, Mock DL, et al: Oral transmucosal fentanyl citrate (lollipop) premedication in human volunteers. Anesth Analg 69:21-7, 1989

30. Lind GH, Marcus MA, Ashburn MA, et al: Oral transmucosal fentanyl citrate for analgesia and anxiolysis in the emergency room. Anesth Analg 70:S241, 1990

31. Ashburn MA, Fine PG, Stanley TH: Oral transmucosal fentanyl citrate for the treatment of breakthrough cancer pain: a case report. Anesthesiology 71:615-7, 1989

32.   Ashburn MA, Olson L, Fine PF, et al: The clinical evaluation of the compassionate use of oral transmucosal fentanyl citrate (OTFC) for the treatment of breakthrough cancer pain (abstract). Pain 5:S353, 1990

33.   Bangham Ad: Introduction. In Liposomes: From Physical Structure to Therapeutic Applications, Knight (ed), Elsevier North-Holland Biomedical Press. The Hague, Chpt 1. 1981

34.   Bangham AD: Liposomes in Nuce. Biol Cell 47:1-10, 1983

35.   Bartholini G, Pletocher A: Cerebral accumulation and metabolism of C14-Copa after selective inhibition of peripheral decarboxylase. J Pharmacol Exp Ther 161:14-220, 1968

36.   Cammon D, Hendee WR, Davis KA: Clinical applications of magnetic resonance imaging -- current status. W J Med 143:793-803, 1985

37.   Chan L: The current status of magnetic resonance spectroscopy-Basic and clinical aspects. W J Med 143:773-81, 1985

38.   Chen G, Ensoi CR, Bohner B: Drug effects on the disposition of active biogenic amines in the CNS. Life Sci 7:1063-74, 1968

39.   De Castro J, Van de Water A, Wouters L, Xhonneux R, Reneman R, Kay B: Comparative study of cardiovascular neurological and metabolic side effects of eight narcotics in dogs. Acta Anaesthesiology Belg 30:5-99, 1979

40.   Dixon JA, Gilbertson JJ: Cutaneous laser therapy. W J Med 143:745-50, 1985

41.   Haigler HJ, Adhojanian GK: Serotonin receptors in the brain. Fed Proc 36:2159-64, 1977

42.   Haveman U, Kuschinsky K: Neurochemical aspects of the opioid induced catatonia. Neurochem Inter 4:199-215, 1982

43.   Haveman U, Turski L, Schwaz M, Kuschinsky K: On the role of GABA-ergic mechanisms in striatum and substantia nigra in mediating muscular rigidity. Naunyn-Schmiedeberg's Arch Pharmac 322 (Suppl):373, 1983

44.   Hause L, Sances A, Larson S: Polarization changes induced in the pyramidal cell and other neural elements by externally applied fields. In the Nervous System and Electrical Currents, Wielfsohn NL and Sances A (ed), Plenum Press, New York, pp 93-95, 1971

45.   Kirkpatrick A, Johansson, Fiserova-Bergerova Y: Ultra-long local anesthesia with lecithin-coated methoxyflurane. Anesthesiology 63:A218, 1985

46.   Knigge KM, Joseph SA, Norton J: Topography of the ACTH-immunoreactive neurons in the basal hypothalamus of the rat brain. Brain Res 216: 333-44, 1981

47.   Kuhan MJ, Pasternak GW: Analgesics: Neurochemical behavioral and clinical perspectives. New York, Raven Press, 1984

48.   Ledue S: L'electrisation cerebrale. Arch Elec Med 11:403-10, 1903

49. Leysen JE, Laduron PM: Receptor binding properties in vitro and in vivo of some long-acting opiates. Arch Int Pharmaco Ther 232:343-6, 1978

50. Leysen JE, Tollenoere JP, Koch MHJ, Laduran P: Differentiation of opiate and neurolept receptor binding in rat brain. Eur J Pharmacol 43:253-67, 1977

51. Martin W: Multiple opioid receptors. Life Sci 28:1547-54, 1981

52. Moore RY, Bloom FE: Central catecholamine neuron systems: anatomy and physiology. Ann Rev Neurosci 1:129-69, 1978

53. Moo-Young GA: Lasers in ophthalmology. W J Med 143:745-50, 1985

54. Myers RD, Oeltgen PR, Spurrier WA: Hibernation 'trigger' injected into brain induces hypothermia and hypophagia in the monkey. Brain Res Bul 7:691-5, 1981

55. Niemegeers CJE, Schellekens KHL, Van Bever WFM, Janssen PAG: Sufentanil a very potent and extremely safe intravenous morphine-like compound in mice, rats and dogs. Drug Res 26:1551-6, 1976

56. Pasternak GW, Childers SR: Opiates, opioid peptides and their receptors. Neurology 31:1311-5, 1981

57. Passternak GW, Childers SR, Snyder SH: Opiate analgesia: evidence for mediation by a subpopulation of opiate receptors. Science May 2:208 (4443):514-6, 1980

58. Pasternak GW, Childers SR, Snyder SH: Naloxazone, a long acting opiate antagonist: effects of analgesia in intact animals and opiate receptor binding in vitro. J Pharmacol Exp Ther 214:455-62, 1980

59. Poznansky MJ, Juliano RL: Biological approaches to the control delivery drugs: a critical review. Pharmacological Rev 36:277-336, 1984

60. Regan JD, Parrish JA: The Science of Photomedicine. Plenum Press, New York, 1982

61. Scherzinger AL, Hendee WR: Basic principles of magnetic resonance imaging. An update. W J Med 143:782-92, 1985

62. Scoggin: The new biomedical technology. West J Med 143:819-24, 1985

63. Sjolund B, Eriksson M: Electro-acupuncture and endogenous morphines. Lancet 2:1085, 1976

64. Snyder SH, Goodman RR: Multiple neurotransmitter receptors. J Neurochem 35:5-15, 1981

65. Standaert FG: Magic bullets, science and medicine. Anesthesiology 63:577-8, 1985

66. Stanley TH, Cazaloa JA, Limoge A, Louville Y: Transcutaneous cranial electrical stimulation increases the potency of N_20 in man. Anesthesiology 57:293-7, 1982

67. Van Bever WFM, Niemegeers CJE, Schellekens KHL, Janssen PAJ: N-4 substituted 1(2-14ylethyl)-4-piperidinyl-N-phenylanamides, a

novel series of extremely potent analgesics with unusually high safety margin. Drug Res 26:1548-51, 1976

68.   Vander Ark GD, McGrath KA: Transcutaneous electrical stimulation in treatment of postoperative pain. Am J Surg 130:338-40, 1975

69.   Verschraegen R, Rossell MT, Bogaert M, Roly G: Maptazind. In: Use in postoperative pain. Acta Anaestheio Belg 27 (Suppl):123-32, 1976

70.   Wofsy D: Strategies for treating autoimmune disease with monoclonal antibodies. W J Med 143:804-9, 1985

71.   Wood PL, Richard JW, Thakur M: Mu opiate isoreceptors: differentiation with kappa agonists. Life Sci 31: 2313-7, 1982

A CONCEPT FOR ASSESSING ANESTHETIC INTERACTIONS

Igor Kissin

According to classic theories of anesthesia based on unitary nonspecific mechanisms of anesthetic actions, one anesthetic may be replaced freely by another, and, in the case of anesthetic combinations, the anesthetic effect of mixtures is expected to be additive (10). However, even if the state of general anesthesia is narrowed to only one of its components and the type of interacting drugs is restricted to inhaled anesthetics, some deviations from additivity can be found (5,7). A rapid increase in the use of intravenous drugs for general anesthesia, especially those acting via specific receptors, is the most important factor requiring revision of the above indicated conceptual approach to anesthetic interactions.

The development of a concept to assess anesthetic interactions is inevitably centered around two major points: 1) identification of the goals of general anesthesia along with the spectrum of pharmacologic actions to achieve them, and 2) determination of the mechanisms of these actions. Although these two aspects of general anesthesia are closely related, they are often discussed separately. The aim of the present article is to combine these aspects in order to better understand the general principles of anesthetic interactions.

STATE OF GENERAL ANESTHESIA AND ITS COMPONENTS

A month after the demonstration of surgical anesthesia by William Morton in 1846, Oliver Holmes suggested the name for it: "The state should, I think, be called anaesthesia" (4). The definition of anesthesia was essentially based on one of the effects of diethyl ether — unconsciousness that provides insensibility in general and to pain in particular. It was soon noted that, in addition to preventing pain, diethyl

T. H. Stanley and T. D. Egan (eds.), Anesthesia for the New Millennium, 153–164.

ether had several other effects that might be useful. Little by little, other useful effects of diethyl ether were also included in the notion of general anesthesia. The effects listed in Table 1 (left side) are commonly provided in anesthesia, all of which are typical for diethyl ether. As a result, general anesthesia was initially accepted as a condition caused by diethyl ether.

According to the classic concept of general anesthesia, the state of general anesthesia is a multi-featured phenomenon with one underlying mechanism, and, to be common for all general anesthetics with diverse chemical structures, this mechanism is supposed to be nonspecific. The problem with the classic concept of the state of anesthesia became obvious when neuromuscular blocking agents, opioids, and barbiturates began to be widely used in combination with inhaled anesthetics. One of the first anesthesiologists to identify the problem was Woodbridge (38). In 1957, he indicated that with the use for anesthesia drugs "having more limited or specific action," the anesthesiologist must "analyze anew what we have been calling anesthesia." He divided anesthesia into four components: sensory blockade; motor blockade; blockade of undesirable reflexes of the respiratory, cardiovascular, or gastrointestinal systems not usually involving the operative field directly; and mental blockade, sleep, or unconsciousness. Different drugs could be used to achieve each component. Woodbridge believed that the initial definition of anesthesia "properly refers to sensory block only"; therefore, he suggested another term to define the state that reflects all four components of anesthesia, "nothria."

Table 2 compares different views on the state of general anesthesia (11,21,27,28,38). Various authors listed (starting from the top of the table) one, two, or more effects in the state of anesthesia. Prys-Roberts (38) indicated that the state of general anesthesia can be defined as "drug-induced unconsciousness, the patient neither perceives nor recalls noxious stimulation." He wrote, "All other attributes of drugs which produce the state of anesthesia can be classed as alternative pharmacological properties of the drugs and not as components of the state of anesthesia." According to the extreme view (presented at the bottom of the table), all separate effects used to protect the patient from the trauma of surgery and induced by one or several drugs should be termed components of anesthesia (21). The authors "do not see any need to reconcile the contradiction between the initial definition of anesthesia with its new meaning by restricting this meaning: all components of anesthesia should be included in the definition of the state of anesthesia. The requirements for different surgeries or patients can be different, dictating appropriate combinations of components of anesthesia." Thus, anesthetic drugs produce effects that, according to the various points of view, can be classified as components of anesthesia or just desirable supplements to anesthesia (Table 1).

Figure 1 compares the hypnotic effect (loss of the righting reflex), blockade of somatic motor responses, and suppression of autonomic responses to noxious stimulation (which might be regarded as basic goals or components of anesthesia) produced in rats with the use of drugs representing different classes of drugs. The comparison shows that each of the representative drugs has its own "fingerprint" of the relationships between the endpoints of anesthesia. The depth of anesthesia can be treated as a passage through ordered stages or planes -- a kind of ordered dose-response curve. With such a curve in mind, the comparison of isoflurane with other agents presented in Figure 1 shows that IV anesthetics are quite different from isoflurane and from one another, and that the passage through different endpoints of anesthesia is far from being similar. For example, thiopental can block the purposeful movement response to noxious stimulation in doses that are far apart from doses that block the cardiac acceleration response. At the same time, these two endpoints can be reached with diazepam at dose levels similar to each other and close to lethal doses. Morphine has the "reversed" ranked order of effects, with loss of the righting reflex at higher doses than blockade of the responses to noxious stimulation. This relationship between components of morphine anesthesia obtained in rat experiments confirms the statement by Hug (19) that some patients with opioid anesthesia may be completely awake and aware of intraoperative events when there is absolutely no change in hemodynamics nor any manifestation of increased sympathetic activity.

Usually, the term "general anesthetic" identifies a drug that can fully provide all components of anesthesia when used alone. With the concept of components of anesthesia, the requirements to classify a drug as an anesthetic become less restrictive. For example, midazolam, which cannot block somatic and cardiovascular responses to noxious stimulation, is regarded as an anesthetic agent.

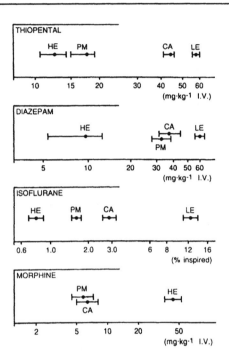

Figure 1. Median effective doses of thiopental, diazepam, isoflurane and morphine for different endpoints of anesthesia in rats. HE=ED$_{50}$ for hypnotic effect (loss of the righting reflex). PM=ED$_{50}$ for blockade of purposeful movement response to noxious stimulation. CA=ED$_{50}$ for suppression of cardiac acceleration response to noxious stimulation. LE=ED$_{50}$ for lethal effect (LD$_{50}$). Horizontal lines=95% confidence limits. From Kissin and Gelman (21).

MECHANISM OF GENERAL ANESTHESIA

Different Drugs Act Via Different Mechanisms

For nearly a century, studies on anesthesia centered on nonspecific, hydrophobic mechanisms of anesthetic action. The fact that general anesthesia is provided by many structurally diverse molecules was usually interpreted as proof that all general anesthetics act via a common nonspecific mechanism. However, extreme diversity of cellular and physiologic mechanisms involved in the anesthetic effect suggest another explanation for this fact: multiple potential neuronal mechanisms that could lead to a common final outcome are likely targets for drugs of dissimilar structure. According to the suggestion by Wall (37), "the apparent similarity of the effect of various anesthetics may not be a reflection of identical modes of action of all anesthetics, but rather a reflection of the varying stability of different synapses."

It is possible to provide general anesthesia with a combination of drugs acting via specific receptors. For example, complete anesthesia can result from the combined use of an opioid, a benzodiazepine, and a neuromuscular blocking drug. All of these drugs act on specific receptors, and their anesthetic effects can be reversed by the administration of specific antagonists. This fact alone makes the unitary hypothesis of anesthetic action unconvincing.

Several attempts have been made to defend the unitary hypothesis by introducing some modifications and by limiting its scope to inhalational anesthetics. For example, the anesthetics acting via the same mechanism can affect more than one molecular site, each of which may have different physical properties — the multi-site hypothesis proposed by Halsey et al. (18). It was realized, however, that the multi-site hypothesis cannot explain much of the evidence against the unitary hypothesis, and Richards (32) postulated that different classes of agents have different mechanisms of anesthetic action.

Franks and Lieb (14) challenged the concept of nonspecific mechanism of anesthetic action and suggested that general anesthetics act by binding to specific molecular sites in the CNS. Recent studies demonstrated a difference in anesthetic potency between the optical isomers of isoflurane (13,25) and also between isomers of etomidate (36). These results represent strong evidence against the nonspecific anesthetic mechanism. In addition, several studies using site-directed mutagenesis showed that mutation of single critical amino acid residue within $GABA_A$ receptor can abolish the effects of enflurane (26) and etomidate (3). This is also an indication that general anesthetics can act via specific mechanisms.

Several possibilities for molecular mechanism of action of general anesthetics are summarized in Table 3. According to this table, each anesthetic at the molecular level can act via one of the following mechanisms: one specific mechanism, a combination of different specific mechanisms, or one nonspecific mechanism. Combinations of some of these mechanisms are also possible (e.g., a combination of specific and nonspecific mechanisms). (For a review on molecular mechanisms of anesthesia, see references 1,8,15.)

As far as the cellular basis of anesthesia is concerned, multiple possible mechanisms have been suggested; these were divided into two major categories, mechanisms involving actions on synaptic transmission and on postsynaptic excitability (for review, see references 17,24,33). Although the CNS synapses have been regarded as the most probable cellular site of anesthetic action (17), other sites and mechanisms are also involved. The anesthetic state may be the result of interactions of multiple different mechanisms that, in combination, provide characteristic behavioral effects.

Different Mechanisms for Different Components of Anesthesia

It was postulated that if different components of anesthesia have the same underlying mechanism of action, general anesthetics should achieve these components in the same proportion. For example, concentrations of different inhaled drugs that are equivalent in terms of preventing movement in response to surgical incision are equipotent in achieving unconsciousness (17). Experiments on animals could not confirm this assumption. Using various inhaled anesthetics in toads, mice, and rats, at least three groups of authors reported that ratios of the ED_{50} values for blockade of noxious stimulation-induced movement to the ED_{50} values for loss of the righting reflex were different with different anesthetics (6,23,34). The initial determination of similar ratios in humans (the ratio of a concentration of an anesthetic that blocks opening of the eyes on command in 50% of patients, MAC-awake, to a concentration that blocks movement to surgical incision, MAC) could not demonstrate a statistically significant difference among them; however, a tendency for a difference between the halothane and the diethyl ether ratios has been observed (Stoelting). Recent clinical studies have reported a difference between MAC-awake/MAC ratios for several anesthetics. In one study (9), the MAC awake/MAC ratio for isoflurane was significantly lower than that for nitrous oxide. The results of another study (16) demonstrated that the MAC awake/MAC ratio for isoflurane (and enflurane) is significantly less than that for halothane. The initial problem of the discrepancy between results obtained in patients and in animal experiments was probably because small differences between various components of anesthesia induced by volatile anesthetics are much easier to detect under laboratory conditions that permit a greater degree of precision.

It is commonly believed that parallel dose-effect curves are indicative of the identity of the mechanism of action. However, the difference in the slopes of dose-effect curves is a less sensitive index for testing the identity of the mechanism of action than agent-to-agent variability in the potency ratios. With inhalational anesthetics, the difference between slopes of the dose-effect curves for different components of anesthesia was reported only for diethyl ether (Kissin et al. 1983). This difference was determined in rats between the slopes of the dose-effect curves for blockade of the righting reflex and for blockade of movement to noxious stimulation. With IV anesthetics, differences between the slopes of the dose-effect curves of an anesthetic for different components of anesthesia are much more pronounced (22).

In 1974, Halsey (17) summarized data indicating the importance of the action of general anesthetics not only on the brain but also on the spinal cord. He wrote that, in animals with a transected cervical spinal cord, the depressant effects of halothane and nitrous oxide on dorsal horn cells equals or exceeds the depressant effect found in animals having intact midbrain and hindbrain cord connections. Recent studies with isoflurane by Rampil (30,31) and Antognini (2) suggest that this drug provides one of the basic components of anesthesia, blockade of movement response to noxious stimulation, by acting primarily on the spinal; cord this occurs at a time when unconsciousness is achieved by the action of isoflurane on the brain. The difference in the anatomic substrate suggests that different physiologic mechanisms are involved in these two actions of isoflurane. Quinlan et al. demonstrated that, in genetically engineered mice, lack of the beta subunit of $GABA_A$ receptor results in a significant difference in the potency of enflurane and halothane for blockade of motor response to noxious stimulation. These data also indicate that different components of general anesthesia can be produced by different mechanisms.

The concept of components of anesthesia resulting from separate pharmacologic actions, even if the anesthesia is produced by one drug, seems to have a sufficient foundation (12,20).

Table 4 reflects changing concepts of the state of general anesthesia.

CONCEPT

When different components of anesthesia are balanced by the combined use of drugs with different mechanisms of action, there is a ground for the wide variability in the anesthetic interaction outcomes (supra-additive, additive, infra-additive) in general. In addition, the same combination of anesthetic drugs could produce different interaction outcomes for different components of anesthesia.

Understanding general anesthesia as a combination of different components achieved through the combined use of drugs with different underlying mechanisms of action has important clinical implications for measuring the depth of anesthesia: different components of anesthesia should be determined specifically for various anesthetic combinations. With the use of anesthetic combinations, the search for a reliable index of anesthetic depth is transformed into a search for separate indices of different components of anesthesia.

TABLE 1. STATE OF GENERAL ANESTHESIA: SPECTRUM OF EFFECTS

Effects	Options to Classify
• Amnesia	• Components of GA*
• Analgesia	• Desirable supplements of GA
• Unconsciousness	• Side effects of GA
• Absence of movement to noxious stimulation	
• Myorelaxation	
• Attenuation of autonomic responses to noxious stimulation	

* GA - general anesthesia

161

TABLE 2. DEFINITIONS OF STATE OF ANESTHESIA

Authors	Definition	Reference
Prys-Roberts	Drug-induced unconsciousness; the patient neither perceives nor recalls noxious stimulation	7
Eger	Reversible oblivion and immobility	8
Pinsker	Paralysis, unconsciousness, and the attenuation of the stress response	9
Woodridge	Sensory block, motor block, blocking of reflexes, and mental block	6
Kissin and Gelman	All separate effects used to protect the patient from the trauma of surgery	10

TABLE 3. POSSIBLE MOLECULAR MECHANISMS PROVIDING MULTIFACETED FEATURE OF ANESTHETIC ACTION

1. One Specific Mechanism

    The spectrum of different effects is achieved by affecting a network element that is crucial for the functions of various CNS systems (e.g., an agent with a specific mechanism of action on the $GABA_A$ receptor complex)

2. Multiple Specific Mechanisms

    The multifaceted outcome is due to a combination of various specific interactions (e.g., an agent that interacts differently with various synaptic channel proteins)

3. One Nonspecific Mechanism

    The spectrum of various effects is achieved by a nonspecific action on an element common to all CNS systems (e.g., an agent disordering membrane lipid bilayers)

TABLE 4. STATE OF GENERAL ANESTHESIA: CHANGING CONCEPTS

General anesthesia represents:

Σ One effect

Σ Several effects with one underlying mechanism of action

Σ Spectrum of effects (components of anesthesia) with different underlying mechanisms for different drugs

Σ Combination of various components of anesthesia resulting from separate

162

pharmacological actions, even if the anesthesia is produced by one drug

REFERENCES

1. Alifimoff JK, Miller KW: Mechanisms of action of general anesthetic agents. In: Rogers MC et al., eds. Principles and practice of anesthesiology. St. Louis: Mosby, 1993:1034-52
2. Antognini JF, Schwartz K: Exaggerated anesthetic requirements in the preferentially anesthetized brain. Anesthesiology 1993;79:1244-9
3. Belelli D, Lambert JJ, Peters JA, et al: The interaction of the general anesthetic etomidate with the g-aminobutyric acid type A receptor is influenced by a single amino acid. Proc Natl Acad Sci USA 1997;94:11031-6
4. Cohen PJ: History and theories of general anesthesia. In: Goodman LS and Gilman A, eds. The pharmacological basis of therapeutics. 5th ed. New York: MacMillan Publishing Co., 1975: 53-9
5. Cole DJ, Kalichman MW, Shapiro HM, Drummond JC: The non linear potency of sub-MAC concentrations of nitrous oxide in decreasing the anesthetic requirement of enflurane, halothane, and isoflurane in rats. Anesthesiology 1990;73:93-9
6. Deady J, Koblin DD, Eger EI II, et al: Anesthetic potencies and the unitary theory of narcosis. Anesth Analg 1981;60:380-386
7. DiFazio CA, Brown RE, Ball CG, et al: Additive effects of anesthetics and theories of anesthesia. Anesthesiology 1972;36:57-63
8. Dluzewski AR, Halsey MJ, Simmonds AC: Membrane interactions with general and local anesthetics: A review of molecular hypothesis of anesthesia. Molec Aspect Med 1983;6:459-83
9. Dwyer R, Bennett HL, Eger EI II, Heilbron D: Effect of isoflurane and nitrous oxide in subanesthetic concentrations on memory and responsiveness in volunteers. Anesthesiology 1992;77:888-98
10. Eger EI II: Does 1+1=2? (Editorial) Anesth Analg 1989;68:551-2
11. Eger EI II: What is general anesthetic action? Anesth Analg 1993;77:408
12. Eger EI II, Koblin DD, Harris RA, et al: Hypothesis inhaled anesthetics produce immobility and amnesia by different mechanisms at different sites. Anesth Analg 1997; 84:915-8
13. Eger EI II, Koblin DD, Laster MJ, et al: Minimum alveolar anesthetic concentration values for the enantiomers of isoflurane differ minimally. Anesth Analg 1997;85:188-92
14. Franks NP, Lieb WR: Do general anaesthetics act by competitive binding to specific receptors? Nature 1984;310:599-601
15. Franks NP, Lieb WR: Molecular and cellular mechanisms of general anesthetics. Nature 1994;367:607-14

16. Gaumann DM, Mustaki JP, Tassonyi E: MAC-awake of isoflurane, enflurane, and halothane evaluated by slow and fast alveolar washout. Br J Anaesth 1992;68:81-4

17. Halsey MJ: Mechanisms of general anesthesia. In: Eger EI II, ed. Anesthetic uptake and action. Baltimore: Williams and Wilkins Co., 1974:45-76

18. Halsey MJ, Green CJ, Wardley-Smith B: Renaissance of non unitary molecular mechanisms of general anesthesia. In: Find R, ed. Molecular mechanisms of anesthesia (Progress in anesthesiology, vol. 2). New York: Raven Press, 1980: 273-83

19. Hug Jr CC: Does opioid anesthesia exist? (Editorial) Anesthesiology 1990;73:1-4

20. Kissin I: General anesthetic action: an obsolete notion? Anesth Analg 1993;76:215-18

21. Kissin I, Gelman S: Components of anaesthesia. Br J Anaesth 1988;61:237-42

22. Kissin I, McGee T, Smith LR: The indices of potency for intravenous anaesthetics. Can Anaesth Soc J 1981;28:585-90

23. Kissin I, Morgan PL, Smith LR: Anesthetic potencies of isoflurane, halothane and diethyl ether for various endpoints of anesthesia. Anesthesiology 1983;58:88-92

24. Krnjevic K: Cellular mechanisms of anesthesia. Ann NY Acad Sci 1991;625:1-16

25. Lysko GS, Robinson JL, Casto R, Ferrone RA: The stereospecific effects of isoflurane isomers in vivo. Eur J Pharmacol 1994; 263:25-9

26. Mihic SJ, Ye Q, Wick M, et al: Sites of alcohol and volatile anaesthetic action on $GABA_A$ and glycine receptors. Nature 1997; 389:385-9

27. Pinsker MC: Anesthesia: a pragmatic construct. Anesth Analg 1986;65:819-20

28. Prys-Roberts C: Anaesthesia: A practical or impractical construct? Br J Anaesth 1987;59:1341-5

29. Quinlan JJ, Homanics GE, Firestone, LL: Anesthesia sensitivity in mice that lack the b3 subunit of the g-aminobutyric acid type A receptor. Anesth Analg 1998; 88:775-80

30. Rampil IJ: Anesthetic potency is not altered after hypothermic spinal cord transection in rats. Anesthesiology 1994;80:606-10

31. Rampil IJ, Mason P, Singh H: Anesthetic potency (MAC) is independent of forebrain structures in the rat. Anesthesiology 1993;78:707-12

32. Richards CD: In search of anesthesia. Trends Neurol Sci 1980;3:9-13

33. Richards CD: The synaptic basis of general anaesthesia. Eur J Anaesthesiol 1995;12:5-19

34. Shim CY, Anderson NB: Minimum alveolar concentration and dose-response curves in anesthesia. Anesthesiology 1972;36:146-51

35. Stanski DR. Monitoring depth of anesthesia. In: Miller RD, ed. Anesthesia, 4th ed. New York: Churchill Livingstone, 1994: 1127-59

36. Tomlin SL, Jenkins A, Lieb WR, Franks NP: Steroselective effects etomidate optical isomers on gamma-aminobutyric acid type A receptors and animals. Anesthesiology 1998; 88:708-17

37. Wall PD: Mechanisms of general anesthesia. Anesthesiology 1967;28:46-51

38. Woodbridge PD: Changing concepts concerning depth of anesthesia. Anesthesiology 1957;18:536-50

DRUG INTERACTIONS:
OPIOIDS AND SEDATIVE HYPNOTICS

Carl Rosow

INTRODUCTION

Modern anesthetic techniques depend heavily on certain drug interactions for safe and predictable induction, maintenance, and recovery. The mixture of an opioid with a true sedative-hypnotic agent (viz., a benzodiazepine, barbiturate, or propofol) is probably the most common combination used in clinical anesthesia. These synergistic interactions can be used to smooth induction, reduce total drug dosage, and decrease side effects. Unfortunately, they can also produce substantial morbidity when unexpectedly intense effects are produced by clinicians who are not prepared to deal with them. This happened when opioid-midazolam combinations were first used by non-anesthesia personnel for endoscopies and radiologic procedures. The unexpectedly large sedative and ventilatory effects led to numerous deaths (1).

DEFINING THE INTERACTION

There is now a rather voluminous literature describing the effects of opioids combined with various induction agents or premedicants. In most cases an additive or synergistic interaction is the result. For example, Ben-Shlomo et al. studied the loss of response to voice in patients given midazolam and fentanyl (2). They found that the hypnotic dose-response curve for midazolam was shifted to the left by a small bolus dose of fentanyl. When the data were analyzed by isobolographic analysis or fractional analysis, the interaction was found to be significantly supra-additive (synergistic). This basic design has been used in numerous

T. H. Stanley and T. D. Egan (eds.), Anesthesia for the New Millennium, 165–170.

subsequent studies. It is an excellent way to quantitate drug interactions, but it is useful to remind ourselves of its limitations:

1. A simple bolus dose-effect design does not allow us to distinguish *pharmacokinetic* from *pharmacodynamic* interaction. In theory, fentanyl could have increased the sensitivity to midazolam by altering its receptor binding, signal transduction, etc. Alternatively, it could have increased the concentration of midazolam by displacing it from protein binding sites, reducing its hepatic metabolism or slowing its renal clearance.

2. The findings do not necessarily apply to other clinical endpoints. For example, the interaction might not have been synergistic if analgesia had been measured.

3. The degree of synergism is specific to the doses tested and the time of testing following the bolus. The results might have been substantially different if the two drugs were given in a different ratio, or the effect was measured at a different time.

CLINICAL IMPLICATIONS

Whether synergistic or additive, opioid-hypnotic combinations are almost always in the direction of increasing CNS depression, and this has important clinical implications. Fentanyl and alfentanil have been shown to reduce the overall requirement for hypnotics such as thiobarbiturates and propofol during short procedures (3,4). In these studies, reducing the total dose of thiamylal or thiopental decreased the time needed for patients to become oriented postoperatively.

Even though the same type of interaction occurs between opioids and propofol, it has been more difficult to show that "propofol sparing" produces an improvement in recovery. Short et al. showed that a combination of alfentanil and propofol reduced the expected propofol ED50 by 20% (5). Thomas et al. found that in short outpatient cases, premedication with 100 mg of fentanyl decreased the requirement for propofol and shortened induction time (6). However, these investigators did not observe any improvement in recovery time or subjective assessment of the quality of anesthesia. This finding may simply reflect the fact that the surgical procedures were extremely brief and the total dose of propofol was low to begin with.

As stated previously, a supra-additive interaction has been demonstrated for opioids and benzodiazepines. This important combination is used for conscious sedation as well as general anesthesia. The hypnotic properties of opioids are relatively weak since even "cardiac" doses of fentanyl and its analogues by themselves do not always produce sleep. We have shown that small doses of diazepam can markedly increase the ability of "high-dose" (100-200 mg/kg) alfentanil to induce hypnosis (7). Similar data are available for hypnosis produced by midazolam with high doses of fentanyl (8). The sedative interaction of midazolam and butorphanol can also be profound (9). Of course, benzodiazepines also markedly increase the vasodilation and respiratory depression produced by opioid agonists (1,9,10).

It is equally interesting if we reverse the perspective and consider the effect of a small dose of opioid on benzodiazepine-induced hypnosis or sedation. A 3 mg/kg dose of alfentanil, by itself, is subanalgesic and subhypnotic (only 2% of the calculated ED50 for unconsciousness), but it can produce a 50% reduction in the hypnotic ED50 of midazolam (11). This means that doses of opioid relevant to the outpatient setting (e.g., 50 mg fentanyl, 500 mg alfentanil) may have very little hypnotic effect alone, but they can effectively potentiate hypnotic drugs used concomitantly. This finding also suggests that when we administer fentanyl plus midazolam for conscious sedation, the opioid is useful for its sedative effects as well as its analgesia.

STUDIES WITH TARGET-CONTROLLED INFUSIONS

More recent studies of opioid-hypnotic interaction have utilized target controlled infusions. This study design has several advantages:

1. If the two drugs are infused for a sufficient time, plasma and effect site concentrations are in rough equilibrium.

2. The exact timing of measurements becomes much less critical.

3. Relating the effect to a measured drug concentration (instead of a dose) minimizes or eliminates the effect of pharmacokinetic variability between subjects.

Fragen has studied interactions during total intravenous anesthesia (TIVA) with remifentanil and propofol (12). The opioid tremendously reduced the infusion rate of propofol needed to suppress movement in response to skin incision (Table 1). Target effect-site concentrations of only 1-2 mg/ml of propofol produced adequate anesthesia in many cases. This is a concentration routinely achieved with propofol doses normally used for conscious sedation (25-50 mg/kg/min). Since the endpoint is movement, this study is comparable to the many studies demonstrating that opioids reduce the minimum alveolar concentration of volatile anesthetics.

A more comprehensive study was conducted by Smith et al. (13) who gave patients target-controlled infusions of fentanyl (0.2 - 4.5 ng/ml) and propofol (1.0-19 mg/ml). These investigators found that fentanyl produced a significant decrease in the amount of propofol needed for unconsciousness (lack of response to voice) and analgesia (lack of movement response to skin incision). The Cp50 for propofol alone (plasma concentration at which 50% of patients respond) was 3.3 mg/ml for voice and 15.2 mg/ml for incision. A fentanyl concentration of 3 ng/ml decreased these values by 40% and 89%, respectively. The hypnotic interaction thus appears to be much more modest than the analgesic interaction.

Interestingly, the same laboratory published an earlier study of thiopental-fentanyl interaction in which they were unable to demonstrate that a moderate analgesic concentration of fentanyl (1 ng/ml) changed the hypnotic concentration of thiopental (14). It is possible that this simply reflects an inadequate dose of fentanyl. Even if this were so, the results are much less impressive than the profound hypnotic synergy demonstrated for opioids and benzodiazepines (11).

FINAL THOUGHTS

It is clear that almost all general anesthetics must be produced with some sort of drug combination, since no single agent has proven optimal as a complete anesthetic. Even high concentrations of volatile agents may not be adequate to suppress all responses to surgery (15). How is the clinician to decide the optimal combination to use for a particular patient, and how can the decision be made for more than one clinical endpoint? Vuyk and colleagues have demonstrated that rigorous quantitation of any 2-drug plus 2 effect combination is possible (16). They analyzed the interaction between propofol and alfentanil given by infusion and determined the probability of movement response to incision as well as the probability of hypnosis. Most interestingly, these investigators then utilized a computer simulation to show the predicted time required to awaken after a 3-hour infusion with all possible drug combinations in the range tested. As might have been expected, the relationship between the drug concentrations and the time to recover had to be graphed in three dimensions – and it was non-linear. This *tour-de-force* analysis cannot be translated easily to the clinical setting, although this has certainly been tried (17). Its value may be in the clear demonstration that the interactions between drugs involve clinical trade-offs which <u>can</u> be measured and predicted.

Table 1. Remifentanil infusion rates (mg/kg/min) in combination with propofol which prevented responses to intubation and incision in 50% of patients. Propofol was administered by computer-controlled infusion to target three specific effect-site concentrations (12).

	Target Propofol Concentration (mg/ml)		
	1	**2**	**4**
Intubation	0.6	0.3	0.2
Incision	0.4	0.3	0.1

REFERENCES

1. Bailey PL, Pace NL, Ashburn MA, Moll JWB, East KA, Stanley TH: Frequent hypoxemia and apnea after sedation with midazolam and fentanyl. Anesthesiology 1990;73:826-30
2. Ben-Schlomo I, abd-el Khalim H, Ezry J, Zohar S, Tverskoy M: Midazolam acts synergistically with fentanyl for induction of anaesthesia. Br J Anaesth 1990;64:45-7

3.   Epstein B, Levy ML, Thein M, Coakley C: Evaluation of fentanyl as an adjunct to thiopental-nitrous oxide-oxygen anesthesia for short procedures. Anesthesiol Rev 1985;2:24-9

4.   Rosow CE, Latta WB, Keegan CR, Philbin DM: Alfentanil for use in short surgical procedures. In: Estafanous FG (ed): Opioids in Anesthesia. Boston: Butterworth, 1984:93-7

5.   Short TG, Plummer JL, Chui PT: Hypnotic and anaesthetic interactions between midazolam, propofol, and alfentanil. Br J Anaesth 1992;69:162-7

6.   Thomas VL, Sutton DN, Saunders DA: The effect of fentanyl on propofol requirements for day case anaesthesia. Anaesthesia 1988;43(suppl):73-5

7.   Silbert BS, Rosow CE, Keegan CR, et al: The effect of diazepam on induction of anesthesia with alfentanil. Anesth Analg 1986;65:71-7

8.   Bailey PL, Wilbrink J, Zwanikken P, Pace NL, Stanley TH: Anesthetic induction with alfentanil. Anesth Analg 1985;64:48-53

9.   Dershwitz M, Rosow CE, DiBiase PM, Zaslavsky A: Comparison of the sedative effects of butorphanol and midazolam. Anesthesiology 1991;74:717-24

10.   Tomichek RC, Rosow CE, Philbin DM, Moss J, Teplick RS, Schneider RC: Diazepam-fentanyl interaction: hemodynamic and hormonal effects in coronary artery surgery. Anesth Analg 1983;62:881-4

11.   Kissin I, Vinik HR, Castillo R, Bradley EL Jr: Alfentanil potentiates midazolam-induced unconsciousness in subanalgesic doses. Anesth Analg 1990;71-65-9

12.   Fragen RJ, Randel GI, Librojo ES, Clarke MY, Jamerson BD: The interaction of remifentanil and propofol to prevent response to tracheal intubation and the start of surgery for outpatient knee arthroscopy. Anesthesiology 1994;81:A376

13.   Smith C, McEwan AI, Jhaveri R, et al.: The interaction of fentanyl on the Cp50 of propofol for loss of consciousness and skin incision. Anesthesiology 1994;81:820-8

14.   Telford RJ, Glass PSA, Goodman D, Jacobs JR. Fentanyl does not alter the "sleep" plasma concentration of thiopental. Anesth Analg 1992;75:523-9

15.   Zbinden AM, Petersen-Felix S, Thomson DA: Anesthetic depth defined using multiple noxious stimuli during isoflurane/oxygen anesthesia. II. Hemodynamic responses. Anesthesiology 1994;80:261-7

16.   Vuyk J, Lim T, Engbers FHM, Burm AGL, Vletter AA, Bovill JG: The pharmacodynamic interaction of propofol and alfentanil during lower abdominal surgery in female patients. Anesthesiology 1995;83:8-22

17.   Stanski DR, Shafer SL: Quantifying anesthetic drug interaction. Implications for drug dosing. Anesthesiology 1995;83:1-5

INTERACTIONS: GENERAL PRINCIPLES

Igor Kissin

General principles of anesthetic interactions are based primarily on several factors that determine pharmacologic properties of general anesthetics: differences in the mechanisms of actions of various drugs determined by specificity of their action, differences in the mechanisms underlying different components of anesthesia, and varying levels of anesthetic efficacy for various drugs and endpoints of anesthesia.

DIFFERENCES IN MECHANISMS OF ACTIONS OF GENERAL ANESTHETICS PROVIDE BASIS FOR SUPRA- AND INFRA-ADDITIVE INTERACTIONS

Although the principle of additivity in general anesthetic interactions was confirmed in many studies with inhaled anesthetics, it was constantly challenged. When interactions of inhalational anesthetics regarding motor response to noxious stimuli were studied in experimental animals, some deviations from additivity were found, primarily when nitrous oxide was involved (3,4). Small deviations from additivity were also found with the hypnotic component of anesthesia in mice, specifically sulphur hexafluoride-nitrous oxide, argon-nitrous oxide combinations (additive), and sulphur hexafluoride-argon combination (infra-additive) (2). It is interesting that the deviations from additivity with combinations of inhaled anesthetics were always toward some degree of antagonism. Findings of the antagonistic interactions between IV anesthetics are usually related to the antinociceptive components of anesthesia. For example, an infra-additive antinociceptive interaction between midazolam and fentanyl was observed in enflurane-anesthetized

T. H. Stanley and T. D. Egan (eds.), Anesthesia for the New Millennium, 171–179.

dogs when the interaction was determined in terms of enflurane MAC reduction (19).

Supra-additive interactions were reported only with combinations of IV anesthetics. Synergism was reported in studies on rats (with loss of the righting reflex as an index of hypnosis) for the following combinations: alphaxalone-etomidate (17), alphaxalone-methohexital (17), and midazolam-thiopental or pentobarbital (12). Midazolam-thiopental synergism was also found in studies on patients with loss of response to voice command as an index of unconsciousness. In one such study (26) presented in Figure 1, dose-response curves for thiopental, midazolam, and their combination were determined with a probit procedure and compared with an isobolographic analysis. The combined midazolam-thiopental fractional dose was found to be only half of the single-drug fractional dose. In other words, the hypnotic potency of the combination was twice the potency of midazolam. Similar results were reported with the midazolam-methohexital combination (25). The observed synergism could be explained by the ability of barbiturates to modulate benzodiazepine receptors (13).

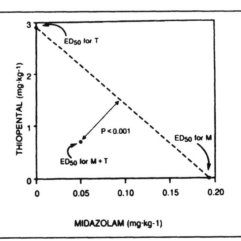

Figure 1. Isobologram for the hypnotic interaction of midazolam and thiopental with the endpoint of loss of the ability to open eyes on verbal command in patients. ED50 values generated by probit analysis indicate the dose level that provides the effect in 50% of patients. T and M are ED50 values for midazolam and thiopental given alone. M + T is the ED50 value for the midazolam-thiopental combination. The dashed straight line connecting the single-drug ED50 points, T and M, is an additive line, and P value indicates the level of statistical significance for deviation of the combined ED50 point to the left of the additive line, indicating a synergism. (From Tverskoy et al.1988)

A synergistic interaction was also reported for the midazolam-propofol combination with the loss of response to verbal command as an endpoint (14,21,27). The hypnotic potency of the combination was found to be 1.5 - 1.7 times the potency of the individual agents.

Benzodiazepine-opioid-hypnotic interactions (loss of response to verbal command) were also found to be synergistic (1,9,22,27). The degree of synergism was reported to be as profound as with the benzodiazepine-barbiturate interactions.

Figure 2 represents the outcome for a triple anesthetic combination: propofol-midazolam-alfentanil. The results of the study reflected by this figure rejected a hypothesis that the triple combination might be even more synergistic than the binary combinations (midazolam-alfentanil, propofol-midazolam, or alfentanil-propofol) due to summation of the binary synergisms (27). The propofol-midazolam-alfentanil interaction produces a profound hypnotic synergism that is not significantly different from that of the binary midazolam-alfentanil combination.

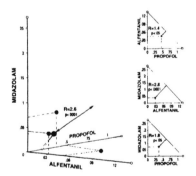

Figure 2. Isobologram for the hypnotic interactions among midazolam alfentanil, and propofol in patients. Shown on the left is a triple interaction, and along the axes, doses of the drugs in mg/kg. The dotted area shows an additive plane passing through three single-drug ED50 points (small open circles); the closed circle, a ED50 point for the triple combination, and the large open circles, ED50 points for the binary combinations. The R-ratio of the single-drug dose (ED50 = 1) to combined fractional dose (in fractions of single-drug ED50 values) reflects the degree of synergism. P value is the significance of the difference from the additive effect. Shown on the right are binary interactions, and dotted lines are additive lines. (From Vinik et al. 1994)

Hypnotic interactions of IV drugs with different mechanisms of actions should not necessarily be non-additive; the best examples are ketamine-thiopental (18) and ketamine-midazolam (6) interactions, which were found to be additive.

The role of the physiologic mechanisms of actions in anesthetic interactions is especially evident in combinations in which an opioid is present. Opioids act as antinociceptive agents, in part by activating the descending inhibitory control systems within the CNS (5). Anesthetics, by inhibiting the descending inhibitory control system, may (in principle) eliminate the supraspinal component of the antinociceptive effect of an opioid and, in addition, the synergism associated with it. For example, a profound morphine-halothane antagonism in relation to suppression of the heart rate increase to noxious stimulation found in rat experiments (11) may be the consequence of such interactions. In these experiments, isobolographic analysis used to characterize the interaction indicated that halothane antagonized morphine to an incomparably greater extent than morphine antagonized halothane.

Thus, there are many examples of non-additive interactions between anesthetics that stem from differences in the nature of their anesthetic actions.

COMPONENTS OF ANESTHESIA AS GROUNDS FOR DIFFERENCES IN ANESTHETIC INTERACTIONS

If components of anesthesia represent separate actions with different underlying mechanisms (even if the anesthesia is produced by one drug), a drug combination may result in different interaction outcomes for different components of anesthesia (8). The most striking illustration for such a possibility is presented in Figure 3. In the study illustrated by this figure (10), the effect of prior administration of reserpine on fentanyl dose-response curves for loss of the righting reflex and prevention of purposeful movement response to noxious stimulation (tail clamping) was determined in rats. Reserpine was found to antagonize the effect of fentanyl on the purposeful movement response and, at the same time, strengthen its effect on the righting reflex. As a result of the reserpine pretreatment, the ranked order for these two effects of fentanyl became the same as with inhaled anesthetics: blockade of the

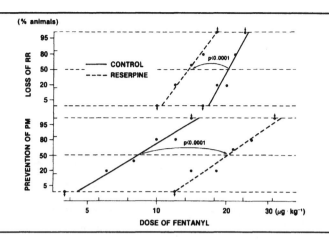

Figure 3. Reserpine-induced changed in fentanyl dose-effect curves for the righting reflex (RR) and purposeful movement (PM) response to noxious stimulation in rats. Along the vertical axis, the percentage of animals (on a probit scale) that reached the specified endpoints. Along the horizontal axis, doses of fentanyl (on a log scale). Each dot represents a group of five animals at the indicated dosage. (From Kissin and Brown, 1985)

motor response occurs after hypnosis. The result suggests that the interaction of intravenous drugs may result in opposite outcomes for different components of anesthesia

Another example, an isobolographic analysis of the morphine-diazepam interactions for the hypnotic effect in rats, demonstrated a profound synergism; at the same time, the morphine-diazepam interaction characterized by abolition of purposeful movement to noxious stimulation resulted in an antagonism (9).

As far as antinociceptive effect is concerned, results similar to those reported in rats were not observed in clinical studies. Although barbiturates in sub-anesthetic doses are known to produce an anti-analgesic effect in humans, this effect is restricted to small doses of barbiturates. When the effects of alfentanil on the hypnotic (verbal command) and antinociceptive (trapezius muscle squeeze) components of thiopental anesthesia were compared in humans, enhancement of the antinociceptive effect of thiopental by alfentanil was even greater than that of the hypnotic effect (9). These results suggest that antagonistic opioid-barbiturate (or opioid-benzodiazepine) antinociceptive interactions might be typical only for rats; they should be regarded only as an indication of the possibility for opposite interactions (synergism versus antagonism) for different components of anesthesia in principle.

Even such close components of anesthesia as inhibition of somatic motor responses and hemodynamic responses to noxious stimulation may not be affected by anesthetic combinations proportionally. For example, in some of the patients anesthetized with a lorazepam-alfentanil combination, somatic responses to noxious stimulation were present at a time when no hemodynamic responses were observed (7).

Thus, a combination of anesthetics can interact differently regarding different components of anesthesia; therefore, some of the combinations that seem advantageous according to the outcome for one component of anesthesia may not be beneficial for another component.

ANESTHETIC EFFICACY

The efficacy of intravenous anesthetics with regard to certain components of anesthesia varies among different agents and can be relatively low. This is especially important for the antinociceptive components of anesthesia. For example, opioid efficacy, in terms of blockade of responses to phasic noxious stimuli, is very low. In the study cited above, Hug and co-authors (7) reported that with a low dose of lorazepam (0.04 mg/kg, premedication) and a very high dose of alfentanil (mean plasma concentration of 2133 ng/ml), seven of nine patients undergoing coronary artery bypass grafting required additional doses of alfentanil to block somatic motor responses to noxious stimulation.

Another illustration of the role of low antinociceptive efficacy of opioids in anesthetic interactions is the so-called ceiling effect. In a dog model in which an opioid was tested as a substitute for an inhalational anesthetic by determination of the MAC value (minimum alveolar concentration of an inhaled anesthetic required to prevent 50 percent of subjects from responding to strong noxious stimulation with gross purposeful movement), it was found that morphine, fentanyl, and sufentanil did not produce a reduction in MAC of enflurane or isoflurane by more than approximately two thirds (16). Similar results were reported with the fentanyl-desflurane (20) and sufentanil-isoflurane (15) interactions in humans. A ceiling effect with a fentanyl-propofol or alfentanil-propofol interaction was also described (23, 28).

The presence of the ceiling effect indicates that the extent of an anesthetic interaction with regard to one of the components of anesthesia is limited, and if the dose of one of the interacting drugs exceeds a certain level, the desired effect will not increase; however, the other effects, which are often detrimental, may continue to increase without such limits.

CONCLUSION

A wide spectrum of pharmacologic actions via different drugs can be used to create the state of general anesthesia. These pharmacologic actions include analgesia, anxiolysis, amnesia, unconsciousness, and suppression of somatic motor, cardiovascular, and hormonal responses to the stimulation of surgery. The spectrum of effects that constitute the state of general anesthesia should not be regarded as several components of anesthesia resulting from one anesthetic action but rather as representing separate pharmacologic actions, even if the anesthesia is produced by only one drug.

Mixtures of agents used to provide anesthesia result in different interactions for different components of anesthesia. Therefore, different components of anesthesia should be determined specifically for various anesthetic combinations and should be considered in anesthetic management (24). With the use of anesthetic combinations, the search for a reliable index of anesthetic depth is transformed into a search for separate indices for different components of anesthesia.

REFERENCES

1. Ben-Shlomo I, Abd-El-Khalim H, Ezry J, et al: Midazolam acts synergistically with fentanyl for induction of anesthesia. Br J Anaesth 1990; 64:45-7
2. Clarke RF, Daniels S, Harrison CB, et al: Potency of mixtures of general anaesthetic agents. Br J Anaesth 1978;50:979-83
3. Cole DJ, Kalichman MW, Shapiro HM, Drummond JC: The non linear potency of sub-MAC concentrations of nitrous oxide in decreasing the anesthetic requirement of enflurane, halothane, and isoflurane in rats. Anesthesiology 1990;73:93-9
4. DiFazio CA, Brown RE, Ball CG, et al: Additive effects of anesthetics and theories of anesthesia. Anesthesiology 1972;36:57-63

178

5. Hanaoka K, Ohtani M, Toyooka M, et al: The relative contribution of direct and supraspinal descending effects upon spinal mechanisms of morphine and analgesia. J Pharmacol Exp Ther 1978;207:476-84

6. Hong W, Short TG, Hui WC: Hypnotic and anesthetic interactions between ketamine and midazolam in female patients. Anesthesiology 1993;73:1227-32

7. Hug Jr CC, Hall RI, Angert KC, et al: Alfentanil plasma concentrations vs. effect relationships in cardiac surgical patients. Br J Anesth 1988;61:435-41

8. Kissin I: General anesthetic action: an obsolete notion? (Editorial) Anesth Analg 1993;76:215-8

9. Kissin I: Interactions of intravenous anaesthetics: general principles. Anaesth Pharmacol Rev 1995;3:90-101

10. Kissin I, Brown PT: Reserpine-induced changes in anesthetic action of fentanyl. Anesthesiology 1985; 62:597-600

11. Kissin I, Kerr CR, Smith R: Morphine-halothane interaction in rats. Anesthesiology 1984; 60: 553-61

12. Kissin I, Mason JO III, Bradley Jr EL: Pentobarbital and thiopental anesthetic interactions with midazolam. Anesthesiology 1987; 67:26-31

13. Leeb-Lundberg F, Snowman A, Olsen RW: Barbiturate receptors are coupled to benzodiazepine receptors. Proc Natl Acad Sci USA 1980; 77:7468-74

14. McClune S, McKay AC, Wright PMC, Patterson CC, Clarke RSJ: Synergistic interaction between midazolam and propofol. Br J Anaesth 1992; 69:240-5

15. McEwan AI, Smith C, Dyar O, et al: Isoflurane minimum alveolar concentration reduction by fentanyl. Anesthesiology 1993;78:864-9

16. Murphy MR, Hug Jr CC: The anesthetic potency of fentanyl in terms of its reduction of enflurane MAC. Anesthesiology 1982;57:485-8

17. Richards CD, White AE: Additive and non-additive effects of mixtures of short-acting intravenous anaesthetic agents and their significance for theories of anaesthesia. Br J Pharmacol 1981;74:161-70

18. Royblat L, Katz J, Rozentsveig V, et al: Anaesthetic interaction between thiopentone and ketamine. Eur J Anaesthesiol 1992; 9:307-12

19. Schwieger IM, Hall RI, Hug Jr CC: Less than additive antinociceptive interaction between midazolam and fentanyl in enflurane-anesthetized dogs. Anesthesiology 1991;74:1060-6

20. Sebel PS, Glass PSA, Fletcher JE, et al: Reduction of MAC of desflurane with fentanyl. Anesthesiology 1992;76:52-9

21. Short TG, Chui PT: Propofol and midazolam act synergistically in combination. Br J Anaesth 1991; 67:539-45

22. Short TG, Plummer JL, Chui PT: Hypnotic and anaesthetic interactions between midazolam, propofol, and alfentanil. Br J Anaesth 1992; 69:162-7

23. Smith C, McEwan AI, Jhaveri R, et al: The interaction of fentanyl on the Cp50 of propofol for loss of consciousness and skin incision. Anesthesiology 1994;81:820-8
24. Stanski DR: Monitoring depth of anesthesia. In: Miller RD, ed. Anesthesia, 4th ed. New York: Churchill Livingstone, 1994:1127-59
25. Tverskoy M, Ben-Shlomo I, Ezry J, et al: Midazolam acts synergistically with methohexitone for induction of anaesthesia. Br J Anaesth 1989; 63:109-12
26. Tverskoy M, Fleyshman G, Bradley Jr EL, Kissin I: Midazolam-thiopental anesthetic interaction in patients. Anesth Analg 1988; 67:342-5
27. Vinik HR, Bradley Jr EL, Kissin I: Triple anesthetic combination: propofol-midazolam-alfentanil. Anesth Analg 1994; 78:354-8
28. Vuyk J, Lim T, Engbers F, et al: The pharmacodynamic interaction of propofol and alfentanil during lower abdominal surgery in women. Anesthesiology 1995;83:8-22

DRUG INTERACTIONS: OPIOIDS AND INHALED ANESTHETICS

Peter S. A. Glass

The concept of what anesthesia is has changed over the past few years. These changes in the concepts of anesthesia have been generated by studies that have shown movement to a noxious stimulus is a spinal rather than cortical reflex (1,2), the effects of volatile anesthetics are probably not related to a nonspecific action but rather they act through specific receptors (3,4), and lastly the results of drug interactions (as described below) imply that inhibition of nociceptive stimuli reaching higher centers of the brain and loss of consciousness play an important role in anesthesia. Thus, to provide the anesthetic state, usually two (hypnotic and opioid) or more drugs are combined. It is well known that one drug may readily alter the disposition (pharmacokinetics) of a second drug. In addition, as the anesthetic state may be produced by drugs acting at a variety of receptor sites, it is not unexpected that their resultant combined effect (pharmacodynamics) will produce complex interactions. The interaction between two volatile anesthetics has been shown to be simply additive; i.e., their combined effect is the result of adding their individual effects (5). However, because of both the pharmacokinetic and pharmacodynamic interactions, when combining intravenous drugs with volatile anesthetic drugs, this simple additive effect is unusual, and a more complex interaction is normally observed.

A pharmacodynamic interaction implies a change in the observed effect when one drug is combined with another, compared to their effect when given alone, and this change in the observed effect is not a result of changes in the drugs' concentration in the biophase (effect) site. Thus, pharmacodynamic interactions exclude interactions occurring as a result of one drug altering the pharmacokinetics of the second drug.

T. H. Stanley and T. D. Egan (eds.), Anesthesia for the New Millennium, 181–194.

Pharmacodynamic interactions occur as a result of several mechanisms most of which are presently ill understood (6,7). At the cellular level, one drug may enhance the binding of a second drug to its receptor or conversely inhibit its binding (e.g., agonist, antagonist). A drug may also alter the intracellular signal transduction pathway of another drug (e.g., the potentiation of the arrhythmogenic effects of beta agonists by volatile anesthetics by both increasing adenyl cyclase activity, or the increased MAC in alcoholics due to development of tolerance of the GABA-ergic receptor), or one drug may effect the uptake or production of neurotransmitters whose release are altered by the second drug (e.g., reversal of neuromuscular blockers by anticholinesterases). A pharmacodynamic interaction may also occur as a result of two drugs acting on two separate receptor systems that share a final common pathway, either at the cellular or subcellular levels. This later mechanism is probably the most common cause for the pharmacodynamic drug interactions seen between drugs used to provide anesthesia.

To establish the concentration of a volatile anesthetic that provides adequate anesthesia, the end-tidal concentration that is in equilibrium with its effect site and will inhibit movement in 50% of patients at skin incision is used (i.e., MAC). To establish the interaction between volatile anesthetics and opioids, the reduction in MAC can be utilized. When performing such studies, it is important that both the volatile anesthetic and the opioid are maintained at stable concentrations and have equilibrated with their effect site. For the volatile anesthetic, this is readily achieved using a calibrated vaporizer. For the opioid, CACI (computer assisted continuous infusion) or similar target controlled delivery devices are used to maintain constant opioid concentration (8).

DRUG INTERACTIONS AND MECHANISMS OF ANESTHESIA

The interaction between fentanyl, sufentanil, alfentanil and remifentanil (analgesics) with either isoflurane, desflurane, sevoflurane (Figure 1B), or propofol (hypnotics) for the prevention of purposeful movement at skin incision is remarkably similar (9-16). There is an initial steep decrease (40-50%) in the MAC/Cp50 with analgesic concentrations of the opiate. Thereafter the decrease in MAC/CP50 with increasing opiate concentration tends to flatten until a ceiling effect is observed. As described by Katoh and Ikeda for sevoflurane and fentanyl (17) (Figure 1A) and Smith et al. for propofol and fentanyl (14) and Vuyk et al. for propofol and alfentanil (15), the interaction for loss of consciousness is very different to that for skin incision with only a 10-20% decrease in the MAC/Cp50 awake value when the hypnotic (propofol or volatile anesthetic) is combined with an analgesic concentration of the opioid.

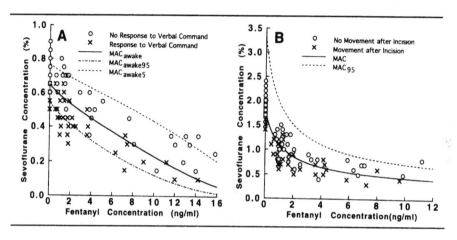

Figure 1 A and B. The interaction between sevoflurane and fentanyl for either loss of consciousness (a) or the prevention of a somatic response at skin incision (B). Note the very different interaction for these two endpoints.

The very different interaction for the two endpoints of loss of consciousness and ablation of a somatic response to a noxious stimulus is strong evidence that loss of consciousness and response to skin incision are not a single continuum of increasing anesthetic depth but rather are two separate phenomena. In addition to preventing a response at skin incision, the minimal concentration of the hypnotic (volatile anesthetic/ or propofol concentration) when combined with a sufficient concentration of opioid is equal to their MAC awake value. It has also been shown that propofol and isoflurane, was alone, require concentrations far in excess of their MAC/Cp50 to prevent an autonomic response to a noxious stimulus, but the addition of analgesic concentrations of fentanyl both inhibits these autonomic responses and reduces the concentration of propofol or isoflurane required (18, 19). If we combine these observations with the fact that the isolated brain requires double the MAC concentration of the intact animal (1), it is possible to propose the following hypothesis of general anesthesia. General anesthesia is a process (Figure 2) whereby a state of

184

STATE OF ANESTHESIA

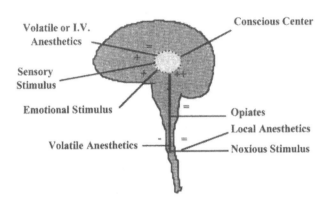

Figure 2. The authors hypothesis of the mechanism for obtaining the state of general anesthesia

unconsciousness of the brain is required (produced primarily by the volatile anesthetic or propofol). When unconsciousness is achieved, a noxious stimulus will cause arousal due to the intensity of the stimulus. To prevent arousal the noxious stimulus needs to be inhibited from reaching higher centers. This is achieved by the action of the opioid at opioid receptors within the spinal cord (or local anesthetics on peripheral nerves, and volatile anesthetics within the spinal cord administered at MAC). If we retain this concept of anesthesia, the drug interactions between volatile anesthetics and opioids make sense and allow the clinician to utilize these interactions to optimize drug administration for anesthesia.

VOLATILE AND OPIOID INTERACTIONS FOR ANESTHESIA

Probably the most commonly used combination of anesthetics is isoflurane and fentanyl. McEwan et al. recently demonstrated that the MAC of isoflurane is reduced markedly by low opioid concentrations (Figure 3 A) (12). A 50% MAC reduction was achieved by 1.7 ng/ml (fentanyl-loading dose of 4 µg/kg followed by 1.75 µg/kg/hr) (5). The minimum effective analgesic concentration of fentanyl is 0.6 ng/ml (20) so that the steepest reduction in MAC occurs within the analgesic concentration range of fentanyl (i.e., 0.5-2ng/ml). Clinically, significant respiratory depression may occur with plasma fentanyl concentrations above 2ng/ml (21). This study by McEwan also demonstrated that beyond 5 ng/ml a plateau or ceiling effect is seen with a maximum MAC reduction of approximately 80%. The maximum reduction in isoflurane was to a concentration of ± 0.3%, close to the MAC awake for isoflurane (22). Alfentanil (16), sufentanil (Figure 3B) (9), and remifentanil (Figure3C) (11) produce similar reductions in isoflurane MAC, with an initial steep

Figure 3. The MAC reduction of isoflurane produced by increasing concentrations of

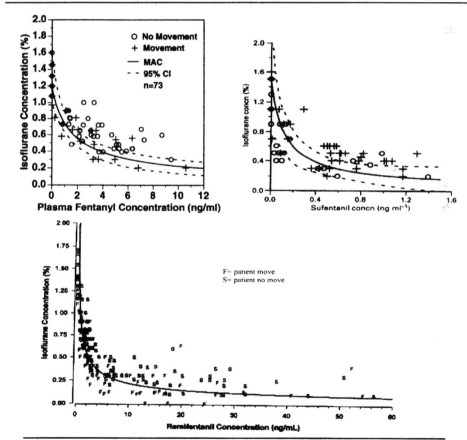

fentanyl (A), sufentanil (B), and remifentanil (C). Note the similar shape of the interaction and the ceiling effect which occurs at an isoflurane concentration of 0.2-0.3%.

reduction at lower concentrations and a plateau effect at higher concentrations. Fentanyl (Figure 3A) (12) and desflurane (13) or sevoflurane (Figure 1) (17) also produce very similar interactions. The concentration producing a 50% reduction of the MAC of isoflurane also provides a means of determining equipotency (in the concentration domain) between the opioids thus far tested (Table 1). Remifentanil is a new esterase metabolized opioid (23-25) which allowed the administration of extremely high concentrations of the opioid. Again, even with this very high concentration (>30 ng/ml), a ceiling effect was still observed with the ceiling at an isoflurane concentration of 0.2-0.3%.

TABLE 1. THE RELATIVE POTENCIES OF THE POTENT μ-SPECIFIC OPIOID AGONISTS BASED ON THEIR ABILITY TO REDUCE THE MAC OF ISOFLURANE BY 50%

Opioid	Plasma Concentration (ng/ml) Resulting in 50% MAC Reduction of Isoflurane	Calculated Potency
Fentanyl	1.57	1
Sufentanil	0.14	12
Alfentanil	28.8*	1/16 (1/55)
Remifentanil	1.37§	1.2

* The 50% MAC reduction of isoflurane by alfentanil was determined following induction of anesthesia with thiopental and thus underestimates the alfentanil concentration
§ Remifentanil was measured as the whole blood concentration
The potency in parentheses is that calculated for alfentanil when corrected for the presence of thiopental.
Reproduced with permission from reference 9.

As stated it would appear that to provide an adequate anesthetic, a minimal concentration of the volatile anesthetic is required to ensure loss of consciousness (i.e., an end-tidal concentration above MAC awake). Of interest is the recent introduction and FDA approval of the bispectral monitor. The bispectral index has been shown to provide a very strong correlation between increasing sedation and loss of consciousness (26) and, thus, may help clinicians titrate the volatile anesthetic to loss of consciousness.

Drug Interactions for Optimizing Drug Dosing

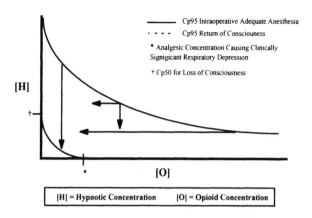

Cp95 Intraoperative Adequate Anesthesia

· · · · Cp95 Return of Consciouness

* Analgesic Concentration Causing Clinically
Signigicant Respiratory Depression

+ Cp50 for Loss of Consciousness

[H]

[O]

| [H] = Hypnotic Concentration | |O| = Opioid Concentration |

Figure 4.   The interaction between volative and opioid to provide adequate intra
operative anesthesia and the decrease in concentration required to return the
patient to the awake state with adequate spontaneous ventilation. The smallest
decrease in either drug concentration occurs when an analgesic concentration of the
opioid is combined with a concentration of the volatile anesthetic just above its
MAC awake concentration.

The above studies on the interaction of opioids with volatile
anesthetics also demonstrate that there is very little advantage in
administering the opioid to higher concentrations once the ceiling effect is
reached.   For fentanyl and remifentanil this is a concentration of
approximately 5 ng/ml, for alfentanil 200 ng/ml, and for sufentanil 0.5
ng/ml.   However, when administering such high opioid concentrations,
recovery from anesthesia and return of spontaneous ventilation may be
markedly delayed.   Thus, the ideal combination of opioid plus volatile
anesthetic is that which provides adequate intra-operative anesthesia and
allows for the most rapid recovery.   As the dose (concentration) of the
opioid markedly affects the amount of volatile anesthetic required to
provide adequate anesthesia, recovery from anesthesia will depend on the
amount of opioid and volatile anesthetic administered, the rate of decrease
of both drugs, and the concentration at which awakening/spontaneous
ventilation occurs (Figure 4).

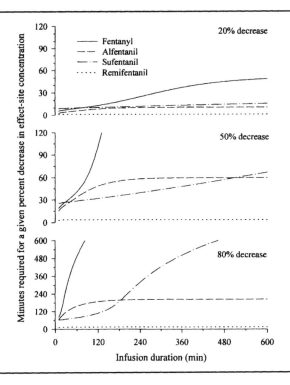

Figure 5. The 20, 50, and 80% context sensitive decrement time for alfentanil, fentanyl, remifentanil, and sufentanil.

Our understanding of the pharmacokinetic processes that determine the recovery from drug effect have also recently been more clearly defined (27,28). The concentration of a drug in the plasma and the biophase is dependent on those processes adding drug to the body and the disposition of drug within the body. When the administration of drug to the body is terminated, the concentration of the drug in the plasma (and biophase) will decrease due to both the irreversible elimination of drug from the body and the redistribution of drug from the plasma to peripheral tissues. Conventional wisdom has been that the elimination half-life of the drug represents the measure of how rapidly recovery from drug occurs. The elimination half-life represents the terminal clearance of the drug and does not incorporate any redistribution of drug and, thus, clearly does not provide any quantitative measure of how long it will take for the drug to decrease by 50%. To provide an estimation of the time for recovery to occur with intravenous anesthetics, the concept of "context-sensitive half-time" was proposed and represents the time required for the plasma concentration of a drug to decrease by 50% (for an infusion designed to maintain a constant concentration) for any given duration of the infusion (28). The context-sensitive half-times for the opioids is shown in Figure 5. It will be noted in Figure 5 that the 'context-sensitive half-time' can vary markedly according to the duration of the infusion: the longer the duration of infusion, the longer the time required for a 50% decrease. The actual percent decrease required at the termination of the procedure to provide awakening and adequate spontaneous ventilation varies according to the dose of opioid administered during the anesthetic. For example, if fentanyl is administered to a concentration of 2ng/ml (loading dose 6 μg/kg followed by 2μg/kg/hr), then only a 30% decrease will be required for adequate spontaneous ventilation. In a similar vein, simulations demonstrate that the time for a 25%, 50%, or 75% decrease in plasma drug concentration is not linear (i.e., a 25% decrease may take 5 minutes, a 50% decrease 20 minutes and a 75% decrease 120 minutes). The context-sensitive decrement times for several different percentage decreases for fentanyl, alfentanil, sufentanil and remifentanil are shown in Figure 5.

Vuyk et al. have performed studies determining the interaction of alfentanil and propofol (15). The results for absence of movement at skin incision with the combination of these two drugs was very similar to that seen with isoflurane and opioids. Vuyk et al. took this interaction one step further in that they also observed the time to awakening at each of these combinations. Thus, not only were they able to define the optimal interaction for the prevention of a response to skin incision, but also the implication of these concentrations on recovery (Figure 6). The differences in recovery time associated with different drugs (i.e., opioid or propofol) was well illustrated in this study. They showed that optimal recovery time occurs at an alfentanil concentration of approximately 80ng/ml and propofol concentration of approximately 3μg/ml. When the concentration of propofol is increased, the concentration of alfentanil can be decreased, but the overall time for recovery increases. Similarly, as the concentration of alfentanil increases, the concentration of propofol can be decreased, but the time for recovery increases. When the concentration of alfentanil is increased beyond 80 ng/ml, even though the concentration of propofol can

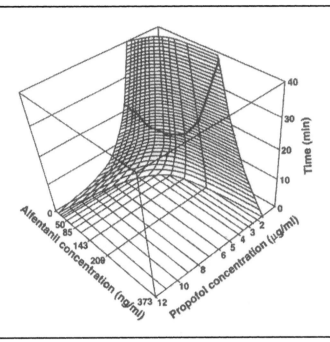

Figure 6. The interaction between propofol and alfentanil for the prevention of
movement at skin incision (x,y axis) and the time for recovery to awakening and
adequate spontaneous ventilation (Z axis) with the combination projected from
the x,y axis.

be reduced there is a marked increase in the time for recovery. This
increase in recovery time is much larger than the increase in recovery time
that occurs when propofol is increased beyond 3µg/ml. A propofol
concentration of 3µg/ml is just above its MAC awake value (14,15). The
recovery profile (offset) of isoflurane is very similar to that of propofol.
Thus, one clinical implication of the drug interaction between volatile
anesthetics with either fentanyl, alfentanil or sufentanil to provide
anesthesia with the most rapid recovery is that the infusion regimen
should provide an analgesic concentration of the opioid equivalent to 1-
2ng/ml of fentanyl (see table 2). The volatile anesthetic should be
administered to the lowest concentration required to provide adequate
anesthesia but to an absolute minimal end-tidal concentration equivalent
to its MAC awake value (e.g., for isoflurane a minimal concentration of
0.3%). If the patient demonstrates signs of inadequate anesthesia, it is
preferable to increase the volatile anesthetic, as increasing these has less of
an effect on prolonging wake-up time than increasing the opioid.

TABLE 2. MANUAL OPIOID INFUSION SCHEMES

Drug	Target Plasma Concentration (ng/ml)	Bolus (ug/kg)	Infusion Rate (ug/kg/min)
Fentanyl	1	3	.020
Fentanyl	4	10	.070
Alfentanil	40	20	0.25
Alfentanil	160	80*	1.00
Sufentanil	.15	.15	0.003
Sufentanil	0.50	.50	0.010
Remifentanil	1	.25	0.025
Remifentanil	5-15	1*	0.2-1.0

* Remifentanil and Alfentanil bolus should given as a rapid infusion over 1-2 minutes.

Remifentanil, as previously stated, has an extremely short context-sensitive half-time of only 3-5 minutes and a context-sensitive 80% decrement time of 10-15 minutes irrespective of the duration of the infusion (Figure 5). This offset is quicker than that achieved with most of the volatile anesthetics. It is preferable to administer remifentanil to high opioid concentrations of 5-12 ng/ml (0.2-0.4µg/kg/min) with just sufficient hypnotic to ensure an unconscious patient. Also, if the patient responds, recovery time is less prolonged by increasing the remifentanil than by increasing the volatile anesthetic. However, it must be reiterated that, although for recovery it is preferable to increase remifentanil, the primary goal is to ensure that the patient is not conscious, and this is only achieved with the volatile anesthetic.

In surgery in which immediate recovery is not required (e.g., most cardiac procedures where post-operative ventilation is planned) and where surgical stimulation is profound, it is probably preferable to administer the opioid to its ceiling effect, thereby ablating any stress response to surgery. In studies in which remifentanil was administered at infusion rates of 1 µg/kg/min, plasma concentrations of epinephrine and norepinephrine (markers of the stress response) were unchanged or decreased from baseline at sternotomy. Thus, for cardiac anesthesia to minimize the stress response and yet provide fast track recovery, it is preferable to use a

192

combination of volatile anesthetic and opioid rather than a pure high dose opioid technique. In this instance, the opioid should be administered at a dose that will be just at the ceiling effect of the opioid (see above). In contrast, in instances in which the patient is expected to breathe spontaneously during surgery, the amount of opioid needs to be limited to avoid significant respiratory depression and higher concentrations of the volatile anesthetic should be used to provide adequate anesthesia. Opioid concentrations should probably not exceed a fentanyl equivalent of 2 ng/ml (3-5 µg/kg loading dose followed by 2 µg/kg/hr).

Anesthesia appears to consist of at least 2 components — analgesia and loss of consciousness. Combining an opioid with a volatile anesthetic achieves this objective. The interaction of volatile anesthetics and opioids in providing anesthesia is complex but consistent. In addition, as 2 drugs are being used to provide anesthesia, recovery to an awake state is dependent on both drugs. Thus, to provide adequate anesthesia and appropriate recovery, it is important to incorporate both the pharmacodynamic interaction that occurs between these drugs as well as their relative offset as demonstrated by their context-sensitive decrement times.

REFERENCES

1. Antognini JF, Schwartz K: Exaggerated anesthetic requirements in the preferentially anesthetized brain. Anesthesiology 79: 1244-9, 1993
2. Rampil IJ: Anesthetic potency (MAC) is not altered after hypothermic spinal cord transection in rats. Anesthesiology 80: 606-10, 1994
3. Tanelian DL, Kosek P, Mody I, McIver MB: The role of the $GABA_A$ receptor/chloride channel complex in anesthesia. Anesthesiology 78: 757-76, 1993
4. Franks NP, Lieb WR: Molecular and cellular mechanisms of general anaesthesia. Nature 367: 807-14, 1994
5. Eger EI, Saidman LJ, Brandstater B: Minimal alveolar anesthetic concentration: A standard of anesthetic potency. Anesthesiology 26: 756-63, 1965
6. Mueller RA, Lundberg DBA: Philosophy and theory, Drug Interactions for Anesthesiology. New York, Churchill Livingstone, 1992, pp 3-19
7. Sear JW: Drug interactions and adverse reactions, Bailliere's Clinical Anaesthesiology, Billiere Tindall, 1991, pp 703-733

8. Glass PSA, Shafer SL, Jacobs JR, Reves JG: Intravenous drug delivery systems, Anesthesia. Edited by Miller R. New York, Churchill Livingstone, 1994, pp 389-416

9. Brunner MD, Braithwaite P, Jhaveri R, McEwan AI, Goodman DK, Smith LR, Glass PS: MAC reduction of isoflurane by sufentanil. Br J Anaesth 72(1): 42-6, 1994

10. Katoh T, Ikeda K: The minimal alveolar concentration (MAC) of sevoflurane in humans. Anesthesiology 66: 301-303, 1987

11. Lang E, Kapila A, Shlugman D, Hoke JF, Sebel PS, Glass PSA: Reduction of isoflurane minimal alveolar concentration by remifentanil. Anesthesiology 85: 721-728, 1996

12. McEwan AI, Smith, C., Dyar, O., Goodman, D., Glass, P.S.A.: Isoflurane MAC reduction by fentanyl. Anesthesiology 78: 864-869, 1993

13. Sebel PS, Glass PSA, Fletcher JE, Murphy MR, Gallagher C, Quill T: Reduction of the MAC of desflurane with fentanyl. Anesthesiology 76: 52-59, 1992

14. Smith C, McEwan AI, Jhaveri R, Wilkinson M, Goodman D, Smith LR, Canada AT, Glass PS: The interaction of fentanyl on the Cp50 of propofol for loss of consciousness and skin incision. Anesthesiology 81(4): 820-8; discussion 26A, 1994

15. Vuyk J, Lim T, Engbers FHM, Burm AGL, Vletter AA, Bovill JG: The pharmacodynamic interaction of propofol and alfentanil during lower abdominal surgery in female patients. Anesthesiology 83: 8-22, 1995

16. Westmoreland CL, Sebel PS, Gropper A: Fentanyl or alfentanil decreases the minimum alveolar anesthetic concentration of isoflurane in surgical patients. Anesth Analg 78(1): 23-8, 1994

17. Katoh T, Ikeda K: The effects of fentanyl on sevoflurane requirements for loss of consciousness and skin incision. Anesthesiology (In press)

18. Kazama T, Ikeda K, Morita K: Reduction by fentanyl of the Cp50 values of propofol and hemodynamic responses to various noxious stimuli. Anesthesiology 87: 213-27, 1997

19. Zbinden AM, Petersen-Felix S, Thomson DA: Anesthetic depth defined using multiple noxious stimuli during isoflurane/oxygen anesthesia II. Hemodynamic responses. Anesthesiology 80: 261-267, 1994

20. Gourlay GK, Kowalski SR, Plummer JL, Cousins MJ, Armstrong PJ: Fentanyl blood concentration analgesic response relationship in the treatment of postoperative pain. Anesth Analg 67: 329-337, 1988

21. Glass PS, Doherty M, Jacobs JR, Goodman D, Smith LR: Plasma concentration of fentanyl, with 70% nitrous oxide, to prevent movement at skin incision. Anesthesiology 78(5): 842-7;, 1993

22. Dwyer R, Bennett HL, Eger EId, Peterson N: Isoflurane anesthesia prevents unconscious learning. Anesth Analg 75: 107-12, 1992

23. Glass PSA, Hardman D, Kamiyama Y, Quill TJ, Marton G, Donn KH, Grosse CM, Hermann D: Preliminary pharmacokinetics and pharmacodynamics of an ultra-short-acting opioid: Remifentanil (GI87084B). Anesth & Analg 77: 1031-40, 1993
24. Egan TD, Lemmens HJM, Fiset P, Hermann DJ, Muir KT, Stanski DR, Shafer SL: The pharmacokinetics of the new short-acting opioid remifentanil (GI87084B) in healthy adult male volunteers. Anesthesiology 79: 881-892, 1993
25. Westmoreland CL, Hoke JF, Sebel PS, Hug CC, Muir KT: Pharmacokinetics of remifentanil (GI87084B) and its major metabolite (GI90291) in patients undergoing elective inpatient surgery. Anesthesiology 79: 893-903, 1993
26. Glass PSA, Bloom M, Kearse L, Rosow C, Sebel PS, Manberg P: Bispectral analysis measures sedation and memory effects of propofol, midazolam, isoflurane and alfentanil in normal volunteers. Anesthesiology 86: 836-847, 1997
27. Shafer SL, Varvel JR: Pharmacokinetics, pharmacodynamics, and rational opioid selection. Anesthesiology 74: 53-63, 1991
28. Hughes R: Interaction of halothane with non-depolarizing neuromuscular blocking drugs in man. Br J Clin Pharmacol 7: 485-490, 1979

AN UPDATE ON THE CLINICAL USE OF PROPOFOL

Paul F. White

Since the introduction of propofol into clinical practice in the late 1980's, over 1000 articles on the intravenous (IV) anesthetic have been published in the peer-reviewed anesthesia literature. Although propofol was initially approved for use as an induction and maintenance hypnotic agent, its clinical uses have expanded greatly to include indications for cardiac, neurosurgical, and pediatric anesthesia, as well as monitored anesthesia care (MAC) and sedation in the intensive care unit (ICU) (1). Propofol has rapidly become the drug of choice for induction of anesthesia in outpatients undergoing ambulatory procedures, and it is becoming increasingly popular for pediatric anesthesia. Propofol's unique antiemetic (2) and mood-altering (3) properties may lead to new clinical applications in the future. Although anecdotal reports suggest that propofol may possess euphorigenic (improved "sense of well-being") properties, this finding has not been substantiated in controlled, double-blind studies (4). Yet, patients clearly "like" the effects of propofol, and it may have potential for abuse or diversion (5).

Information regarding propofol's pharmacokinetic and pharmacodynamic properties has facilitated the use of this drug in clinical practice (6). As expected, patient responses to propofol during the perioperative period vary widely. Therefore, the dosage and rate of propofol administration should be titrated to the needs of the individual patient. Factors that influence propofol dosage requirements include age, weight, preexisting medical conditions, type of surgical procedure, and concomitant medical therapy. As part of a balanced or total intravenous anesthetic (TIVA) technique, infusion rates of 70 to 300 $mg \bullet kg^{-1} \bullet min^{-1}$ are usually required, whereas adequate sedation can be maintained with

T. H. Stanley and T. D. Egan (eds.), Anesthesia for the New Millennium, 195–198.

infusion rates of 25 to 100 $mg \cdot kg^{-1} \cdot min^{-1}$. Anesthesiologists can define "target" plasma concentrations for hypnosis (2 to 6 $\mu g \cdot ml^{-1}$) and sedation (0.5 to 1.5 $\mu g \cdot ml^{-1}$) during a variety of clinical conditions. Pharmacokinetically-based delivery systems can rapidly achieve targeted plasma concentrations of propofol (7). However, careful titration to the desired clinical effect is essential because of the inherent pharmacokinetic and pharmacodynamic variability among patients. In addition, the therapeutic propofol concentration depends on the surgical stimulus (8).

Studies on the molecular mechanism of propofol's effects on the central nervous system (CNS) suggest that, like other CNS depressants (e.g., barbiturates, etomidate), propofol activates the $GABA_A$ receptor-chloride ionophore complex (9). At clinically relevant concentrations, propofol increases chloride conductance. However, at high concentrations of propofol, desensitization of the $GABA_A$ receptor results in suppression of the inhibitory system. The mechanism of propofol's antiemetic activity is yet to be explained.

In addition to discussing information regarding propofol's clinical pharmacologic and physiologic effects, the relevant literature relating to its use in ambulatory, pediatric, cardiac anesthesia and for neuroanesthesia will be reviewed. Clinical applications of propofol infusions for sedation during local and regional anesthesia, as well as outside the operating room (e.g., ICU, radiologic suite), will be discussed.

SUMMARY

Propofol has become a widely used IV anesthetic for induction and maintenance of general anesthesia and for sedation in a wide variety of clinical situations. In patients with asthma, propofol offers significant advantages over the barbiturates for induction of anesthesia (10). The favorable recovery profile associated with propofol offers advantages over traditional anesthetic and sedative medications in clinical situations where rapid recovery is important. The use of propofol in combination with the EEG BIS monitoring device may facilitate an even more rapid emergence and early recovery (11). However, faster recovery will only reduce overall costs if it permits a reduction in manpower or equipment utilization (12). Controversy exists regarding the cost-effectiveness of propofol-based (versus inhalation) anesthetic techniques (12-15). In the future, outcome studies involving propofol should address specific patient populations and should also include an assessment of patient well-being and resumption of normal activities. Although propofol would appear to be an ideal anesthetic for outpatient laparoscopic pronuclear stage transfer (PROST) procedures because of its excellent recovery profile and low incidence of PONV, its use was allegedly associated with lower pregnancy rates compared with isoflurane (16). Further studies are needed in this patient population, as well as in other clinical situations where controversy exists regarding the use of this valuable agent. Although many questions still remain regarding this unique sedative-hypnotic drug, propofol has indeed provided a "new awakening" in anesthesia (17).

REFERENCES

1. Smith I, White PF, Nathanson M, Gouldson R: Propofol: an update on its clinical uses. Anesthesiology 1994;81:1005-43
2. Borgeat A, Wilder-Smith OHG, Saiah M, Rifat K: Sub hypnotic doses of propofol possess direct antiemetic properties. Anesth Analg 1992;74:539-41
3. Zacny JP, Lichtor JL, Coalson DW, et al: Subjective and psychomotor effects of subanesthetic doses of propofol in healthy volunteers. Anesthesiology 1992;76:696-702
4. Whitehead C, Sanders LD, Oldroyd G, et al: The subjective effects of low-dose propofol: a double-blind study to evaluate dimensions of sedation and consciousness with low-dose propofol. Anaesthesia 1994;49:490-6
5. Zacny JP, Lichtor JL, Zarogoza JG: Assessing the behavioral effects and abuse potential of propofol bolus injections in healthy volunteers. Drug Alcohol Depend 1993;32:45-57
6. Shafer SL: Advances in propofol pharmacokinetics and pharmacodynamics. J Clin Anesth 1993;5:14S-21S
7. Kenny GNC: Practical experience with computer-controlled propofol infusion. Semin Anesth 1992;11:12-3
8. Shafer A, Doze VA, Shafer SL, White PF: Pharmacokinetics and pharmacodynamics of propofol infusions during general anesthesia. Anesthesiology 1988;69:456-8
9. Hara M, Kai Y, Ikemoto Y: Propofol activates $GABA_A$ receptor-chloride ionophore complex in dissociated hippocampal pyramidal neurons of the rat. Anesthesiology 1993;79:781-8
10. Pizov R, Brown Rh, Weiss YS, et al: Wheezing during induction of general anesthesia in patients with and without asthma. Anesthesiology 1995;82:1111-6

11. Gan TJ, Glass PS, Windsor A, Payne F, Rosow C, Sebel P, Manberg P and the BIS Utility Study Group: Bispectral index monitoring allow faster emergence and improved recovery from propofol, alfentanil, and nitrous oxide anesthesia. Anesthesiology 1997;87:808-15

12. Watcha MF, White PF: Economics of anesthetic practice. Anesthesiology 1997;86:1170-96

13. Biro P, Suter G, Alon E: Intravenous anesthesia with propofol versus thiopental-enflurane anesthesia: a consumption and cost analysis. Anaesthesist 1995;4:163-70

14. Alhashemi JA, Miller DR, O'Brien HV, Hull KA: Cost-effectiveness of inhalational, balanced and total intravenous anaesthesia for ambulatory knee surgery. Can J Anaesth 1997;44:118-25

15. Boldt J, Jaun N, Kumle B, Heck M, Mund K: Economic considerations of the use of new anesthetics: a comparison of propofol, sevoflurane, desflurane, and isoflurane. Anesth Analg 1998;86:504-9

16. Vincent RD, Syrop CH, Van Voohis BJ, et al: An evaluation of the effect of anesthetic technique on reproductive success after laparoscopic pronuclear stage transfer: propofol/nitrous oxide versus isoflurane/nitrous oxide. Anesthesiology 1995;82:352-8

17. Anonymous: New awakening in anesthesia: at a price. Lancet 1987;1:1469-70

KINETIC CONSIDERATIONS IN THE SELECTION OF AN INHALED ANESTHETIC

Edmond I Eger II

Kinetic profiles of many new anesthetic drugs permit a more rapid and precise adjustment of effect, including a more rapid recovery of normal function. Desflurane and, to a lesser extent, sevoflurane fit this mold. These newest inhaled anesthetics differ kinetically from isoflurane and halothane because of their lower solubility in blood (Table), a feature produced by halogenation solely with fluorine [CHF_2-O-CHF-CF_3 (desflurane); CH_2F-O-CH-$(CF_3)_2$ (sevoflurane)]. Tissue/gas partition coefficients approximately double from desflurane to sevoflurane to isoflurane to halothane (Table).

Human Blood/Gas and Tissue/Gas Partition Coefficients (Mean±SD) (1-4)

Tissue	Desflurane	Sevoflurane	Isoflurane	Halothane
Blood	0.42±0.02	0.69±0.05	1.46±0.09	2.54±0.18
Brain	0.54±0.02	1.2±0.1	2.1±0.1	4.8±0.4
Heart	0.54±0.07	1.2±0.1	2.2±0.3	4.6±0.8
Liver	0.55±0.06	1.2±0.2	2.3±0.3	5.1±0.7
Kidney	0.40±0.05	0.78±0.12	1.4±0.2	2.8±0.5
Muscle	0.94±0.35	2.4±1.0	4.4±2.0	9.5±4.6
Fat	12±2	34±6	64±12	136±33

Comparison of the properties of isoflurane and desflurane illustrates the effect of substitution of fluorine for chlorine. Desflurane differs from isoflurane (CHF_2-O-CHCl-CF_3) only by a fluorine for chlorine substitution. This substitution increases vapor pressure at room temperature (240 mm Hg for isoflurane and 670 mm Hg for desflurane) and decreases potency (MAC for sevoflurane in middle-aged patients is 2%; for desflurane, it is

199

T. H. Stanley and T. D. Egan (eds.), Anesthesia for the New Millennium, 199–206.
© 1999 Kluwer Academic Publishers.

6%, five times the value of 1.15% for isoflurane). MAC-Awake (the concentration permitting voluntary response to command in 50% of patients) is a third of MAC for desflurane and sevoflurane (5-6), as well as for isoflurane (7). This finding is important because MAC-Awake may indicate the concentration providing amnesia as well as the concentration at which awakening occurs. Such data suggest that desflurane and sevoflurane are potent amnestic drugs.

The lower solubility of desflurane and sevoflurane indicates a more rapid rate of rise of the alveolar concentration towards the concentration inspired. Several results confirm this prediction (Figure 1) (8,9). In the case of sevoflurane, the rapidity of change correctly implies a capacity to rapidly induce anesthesia, a rapidity which usually equals that available with halothane (10). However, recent studies in infants and children where the anesthetist was blinded to the choice of anesthetic indicate that 8% sevoflurane does not produce a more rapid induction of anesthesia than 5% halothane (10), and in one report the induction with sevoflurane was slower (11). In contrast to sevoflurane or halothane, the pungency of desflurane at concentrations exceeding 6% results in respiratory tract

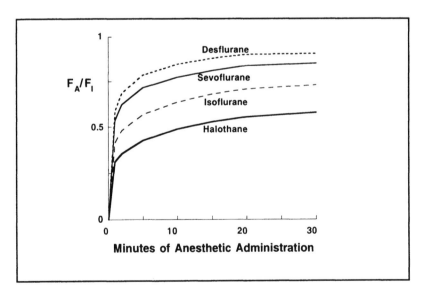

Figure 1. The alveolar concentration (F_A) rises to the inspired concentration (F_I) at a rate inversely related to the solubility of the anesthetic in blood (8,9). Reproduced with permission from Eger (12).

irritation and coughing, breathholding and laryngospasm. These responses limit desflurane's usefulness as an induction agent, and desflurane is not recommended for this purpose, especially in children.

Once induction is complete, the effect of pungency on clinical practice appears to be minor or non-existent. During maintenance, the concentration of desflurane or sevoflurane can be rapidly adjusted to meet changing clinical needs. Furthermore, the difference between the inspired and alveolar concentrations is relatively small, and the inspired concentration may be used as a surrogate of the alveolar concentration. In turn, given a modest inflow rate (1 L/min or greater), the difference between the concentration delivered from the vaporizer and that in inspired gas becomes small (presently, however, sevoflurane is not recommended for use at flow rates less than 2 L/min because of issues of toxicity). Thus, the alveolar concentration and the level of anesthesia may be controlled and known if one uses an accurately calibrated vaporizer and a modest inflow rate. For more soluble anesthetics, the difference between the concentration delivered and that in the alveoli may be considerable.

As would be predicted from their low solubilities, elimination of anesthetic from the body and recovery from anesthesia during the first 10-20 min after anesthesia are faster with sevoflurane and desflurane than with isoflurane (13-15). Immediate and longer-term recovery from desflurane is more rapid than recovery from sevoflurane (Fig. 2) (16). This includes recovery from desflurane versus sevoflurane or halothane anesthesia in infants (17). Regarding stay in the recovery room, a short duration of anesthesia appears to produce limited differences from agents such as isoflurane in long-term recovery (18), but the results of at least three studies suggest a more rapid release after anesthesia with desflurane (19-21). In contrast, studies to date appear not to show a difference in time to discharge after anesthesia with sevoflurane vs. isoflurane (22). To make use of the potential for an earlier release from the recovery room may require the development of new guidelines for the dismissal of patients.

Both sevoflurane and desflurane cost more to purchase than older compounds such as halothane and isoflurane. In dollars per case, the difference will be influenced by the kinetics of the agents used and by the flow rates used. The lower solubilities of desflurane and sevoflurane enhance the ease with which low flow anesthesia may be delivered. For example, at UCSF we commonly use flows of 1 L/min or less with desflurane, providing maintenance of anesthesia at a cost of $2-$4 per hour.

Time from Cessation of Anesthesia to Response to Command and to Orientation to Place and Date

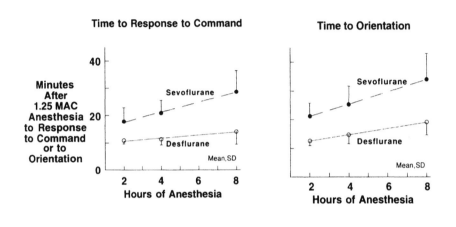

Figure 2. Volunteers anesthetized with desflurane for 2, 4, or 8 hr respond to command sooner and are oriented sooner than the same volunteers after anesthesia with 1.25 MAC sevoflurane (16,23). Reproduced with permission (23).

A similar application with sevoflurane is limited by the present package warning not to use flows less than 2 L/min. The greater cost of desflurane versus isoflurane may also be offset by decreased operating room and PACU costs if advantage is taken of the shorter recovery times possible with this anesthetic.

In an effort to economize yet obtain a rapid recovery, one might consider using the relatively inexpensive isoflurane for the first part of anesthesia and desflurane for the latter portion. We have studied this possibility, finding that the substitution of desflurane for isoflurane during the final half hour of a 2 hour anesthesia, always at 1.25 MAC, does not hasten recovery (Fig. 3) (24).

One element of rapid recovery may be undesirable. Children anesthetized with desflurane or sevoflurane for maintenance of anesthesia may awaken with more excitation than with older, more soluble anesthetics (25). This does not appear to be a problem with adults.

Certain cardiovascular effects may be pertinent to a consideration of induction of anesthesia. Under steady-state conditions in unstimulated adults, sevoflurane and desflurane have similarly minimal effects on heart

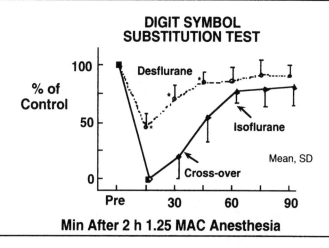

DIGIT SYMBOL SUBSTITUTION TEST

Figure 3. Substitution of desflurane for isoflurane during the last 30 min of a 120 min anesthetic ("crossover") did not accelerate late recovery as measured by digit symbol substitution test (DSST) (P>0.05). Anesthesia for the entire 2 hour period totaled 1.25 MAC (i.e., in the crossover group, desflurane was added as isoflurane was eliminated, at all times producing a total MAC of 1.25). There was no significant difference at any time for recovery of cognitive function between isoflurane and "crossover," but the values for desflurane differed significantly (asterisks) from both isoflurane and "crossover" groups. Return to values not different from the 100% of control occurred for desflurane after 45 min but for isoflurane and "crossover" such recovery occurred after 75 min. Adopted with permission from Neumann et al. (24)

rate and produce similar decreases in blood pressure. In addition, desflurane (and, to a lesser extent, isoflurane) can transiently (3-6 min) increase both pulse rate and blood pressure when the inspired concentration is rapidly increased above MAC (26,27). Fentanyl administration may attenuate these transient increases in heart rate and blood pressure (28). Second and third increases in desflurane concentrations produce only muted increases in rate and pressure (i.e., the initial response to desflurane rapidly adapts) (29). In contrast to the capacity of desflurane to transiently increase heart rate and blood pressure, sevoflurane does not increase heart rate or blood pressure when the concentration is acutely increased above 1 MAC.

In summary, the kinetics of both desflurane and sevoflurane offer advantages over other modern inhaled anesthetics. An absence of pungency allows sevoflurane to be used to induce anesthesia as rapidly as halothane, whereas concentrations of desflurane exceeding 1 MAC have a pungency that hinders induction by inhalation. Both agents (desflurane more than sevoflurane) provide a greater precision of control over anesthetic administration than isoflurane, and both permit a more rapid recovery from anesthesia. The more rapid recovery with desflurane (but not sevoflurane) can lead to an earlier discharge from both the operating room and the PACU.

REFERENCES

1. Eger EI, II: Partition coefficients of I-653 in human blood, saline, and olive oil. Anesth Analg 1987; 66:971-3
2. Strum DP, Eger EI, II: Partition coefficients for sevoflurane in human blood, saline, and olive oil. Anesth Analg 1987; 66:654-6
3. Eger RR, Eger EI, II: Effect of temperature and age on the solubility of enflurane, halothane, isoflurane and methoxyflurane in human blood. Anesth Analg 1985; 64:640-2
4. Yasuda N, Targ AG, Eger EI, II: Solubility of I-653, sevoflurane, isoflurane, and halothane in human tissues. Anesth Analg 1989; 69:370-3
5. Jones RM, Cashman JN, Eger EI, II, Damask MC, Johnson BH: Kinetics and potency of desflurane (I-653) in volunteers. Anesth Analg 1990; 70:3-7
6. Katoh T, Suguro Y, Nakajima R, Kazama T, Ikeda K: Blood concentration of sevoflurane and isoflurane on recovery from anaesthesia. Br J Anaesth 1992; 69:259-62
7. Dwyer R, Bennett HL, Eger EI, II, Heilbron D: Effects of isoflurane and nitrous oxide in subanesthetic concentrations on memory and responsiveness in volunteers. Anesthesiology 1992; 77:888-98
8. Yasuda N, Lockhart SH, Eger EI, II, Weiskopf RB, Liu J, Laster M, Taheri S, Peterson NA: Comparison of kinetics of sevoflurane and isoflurane in humans. Anesth Analg 1991; 72:316-24
9. Holaday DA, Smith FR: Clinical characteristics and biotransformation of sevoflurane in healthy human volunteers. Anesthesiology 1981; 54:100-6
10. Bacher A, Burton AW, Uchida T, Zornow MH: Sevoflurane or halothane anesthesia: Can we tell the difference? Anesth Analg 1997; 85:1203-6

11. O'Brien K, Kumar R, Morton NS: Sevoflurane compared with halthane for tracheal intubation in children. Br J Anaesth 1998; 80:452-5

12. Eger EI, II: Desflurane (Suprane). A Compendium and Reference. Healthpress Publishing Group. Rutherford, NJ. 1993; pp 1-119

13. Eger EI, II, Johnson BH: Rates of awakening from anesthesia with I-653, halothane, isoflurane, and sevoflurane: A test of the effect of anesthetic concentration and duration in rats. Anesth Analg 1987; 66:977-82

14. Ghouri AF, Bodner M, White PF: Recovery profile after desflurane-nitrous oxide versus isoflurane-nitrous oxide in outpatients. Anesthesiology 1991; 74:419-24

15. Frink EJ, Jr, Malan TP, Atlas M, Dominguez LM, DiNardo JA, Brown BR, Jr: Clinical comparison of sevoflurane and isoflurane in healthy patients. Anesth Analg 1992; 74:241-5

16. Eger EI, II, Bowland T, Ionescu P, Laster MJ, Fang ZX, Gong D, Sonner J, Weiskopf RB: Recovery and kinetic characteristics of desflurane and sevoflurane in volunteers after 8-hour exposure, including kinetics of degradation products. Anesthesiology 1997; 87:517-26

17. O'Brien K, Robinson DN, Morton NS: Induction and emergence in infants less than 60 weeks post-conceptual age: comparison of thiopental, halothane, sevoflurane and desflurane. Br J Anaesth 1998; 80:456-9

18. Gupta A, Kullander M, Ekberg K, Lennmarken C: Anaesthesia for day-care arthroscopy. A comparison between desflurane and isoflurane. Anaesthesia 1996; 51:56-62

19. Natonson RA, Anpel LL, Gilbert HC, Ragin A: Comparisons of cost and recovery following desflurane or isoflurane anesthesia. Anesthesiology 1995; 83:A50

20. Bennett JA, Lingaraju N, Horrow JC, McElrath T, Keykhah MM: Elderly patients recover more rapidly from desflurane than from isoflurane anesthesia. J Clin Anesth 1992; 4:378-81

21. Tsai SK, Lee C, Kwan W-F, Chen B-J: Recovery of cognitive functions after anaesthesia with desflurane or isoflurane and nitrous oxide. Br J Anaesth 1992; 69:255-8

22. Philip BK, Kallar SK, Bogetz MS, Scheller MS, Wetchler BV, SMAG: A multicenter comparison of maintenance and recovery with sevoflurane or isoflurane for adult ambulatory anesthesia. Anesth Analg 1996; 83:314-9

23. Eger EI, II, Gong D, Koblin DD, Bowland T, Ionescu P, Laster MJ, Weiskopf RB: Effect of anesthetic duration on kinetic and recovery characteristics of desflurane vs. sevoflurane (plus compound A) in volunteers. Anesth Analg 1998; 86:414-21

24. Neumann MA, Weiskopf RB, Gong DH, Eger EI, II, Ionescu P: Changing from isoflurane to desflurane towards the end of anesthesia

does not accelerate recovery in humans. Anesthesiology 1998; 88:(In press)

25. Aono J, Ueda W, Mamiya K, Takimoto E, Manabe M: Greater incidence of delirium during recovery from sevoflurane anesthesia in preschool boys. Anesthesiology 1997; 87:1298-300

26. Ebert TJ, Muzi M: Sympathetic hyperactivity during desflurane anesthesia in healthy volunteers. A comparison with isoflurane. Anesthesiology 1993; 79:444-53

27. Weiskopf RB, Moore M, Eger EI, II, M MN, McKay L, Chortkoff BS, Hart PS, Damask M: Rapid increase in desflurane concentration is associated with greater transient cardiovascular stimulation than with rapid increase in isoflurane concentration in humans. Anesthesiology 1994; 80:1035-45

28. Weiskopf RB, Eger EI, II, Noorani M, Daniel M: Fentanyl, esmolol, and clonidine blunt the transient cardiovascular stimulation induced by desflurane in humans. Anesthesiology 1994; 81:1350-5

29. Weiskopf RB, Eger EI, II, Noorani M, Daniel M: Repetitive rapid increases in desflurane concentration blunt transient cardiovascular stimulation in humans. Anesthesiology 1994; 81:843-9

CONTROVERSIES REGARDING SEVOFLURANE & DESFLURANE TOXICITY

Edmond I Eger II

The new anesthetics, desflurane and sevoflurane, differ from their predecessors in that these new anesthetics are halogenated solely with fluorine. The absence of chlorine and bromine increases the stability of these anesthetics, but the increased stability is not perfect. Thus, we need to consider the potential of each to be metabolized in the body or degraded by strong base (carbon dioxide absorbents) into toxic compounds.

Desflurane and sevoflurane differ in their resistance to biodegradation. Desflurane resists biodegradation. Degradation is too small to measure accurately. Approximately 0.02% of the desflurane taken up during its administration can be recovered as urinary metabolites (1). The metabolism of sevoflurane is approximately 100 times greater (2), slightly exceeding that of enflurane. Inorganic fluoride and trifluoroacetate result from the metabolism of desflurane. Inorganic fluoride, formic acid, and hexafluoroisopropanol result from the metabolism of sevoflurane.

Anesthetic biodegradation is of concern because of the link between degradation and toxicity observed with several older anesthetics such as chloroform, methoxyflurane, halothane, and possibly enflurane. By this reasoning, desflurane should be minimally toxic, and results from studies in animals and 20 million humans bear out this prediction. Because of its metabolism, sevoflurane is less above suspicion. However, extensive studies in animals and humans reveal limited evidence of toxicity. Sevoflurane has also been used in 20 million patients with few reports of clinically significant injury. One report found transient impairment of renal function after prolonged sevoflurane anesthesia (3), and based on this and other reports, Mazze and Jamison recommended that sevoflurane not be used in patients with impaired renal function (4). Goldberg et al. found

T. H. Stanley and T. D. Egan (eds.), Anesthesia for the New Millennium, 207–212.
© 1999 *Kluwer Academic Publishers.*

increases in creatinine and BUN in a few patients anesthetized for longer (approximately 3 hr) intraabdominal procedures with sevoflurane, particularly in association with higher concentrations of inorganic fluoride (5). Although comparable patients in this study given isoflurane did not have increases in creatinine or BUN, the results for sevoflurane may have been confounded by factors such as the site of surgery and dehydration.

The strength of the carbon-fluorine bond increases physical stability, a fortunate effect because alkali (e.g., Baralyme®) degrade sevoflurane, especially at the increased temperatures found in the carbon dioxide absorber needed for closed circuit anesthesia. Were its stability less, sevoflurane might not be clinically useful. In contrast, desflurane resists degradation by standard absorbents (those containing a normal compliment of water) and does so more than its chlorinated analog, isoflurane. Sevoflurane breaks down into a lethal product [CFH_2-O-C(=CF_2)(CF_3), also known as compound A] that in clinical practice (6,7) appears in concentrations associated with injury in rats (6,8,9). Biochemical abnormalities in rats coincide with the appearance in the same rats of histological evidence of change, specifically renal necrosis (10). Similarly, Cynomolgus monkeys that breathe 100 ppm compound A for 8 hours have increased urinary protein and N-acetyl glucosaminidase as well as single cell necrosis and tubular degeneration (11). These findings raise concern that through its degradation to compound A, sevoflurane may injure human kidneys (12). In volunteers, anesthesia with 1.25 MAC sevoflurane for 8 hours can produce average compound A concentrations of 40 ppm and associated transient renal damage as revealed by increases in urinary albumin, glucose and the tubular enzyme a-GST (13). The same volunteers show no significant abnormalities in these variables when given desflurane for comparable periods and concentrations. More recently we demonstrated that a 4-hr anesthetic with sevoflurane at 1.25 MAC can cause renal injury in volunteers (14). In contrast, Bito et al. (15) and Kharasch et al. (16) found no difference in the injurious effects of sevoflurane vs. isoflurane in patients. These apparently discrepant findings can be reconciled by the concept of a threshold; our data were obtained at doses of compound A (ppm-hr) that exceeded 150 ppm-hr, whereas Bito et al. applied a dose of 122 ppm-hr and Kharasch et al. a dose of 79 ppm-hr. More recent results document that compound A can cause renal injury in humans (17,18). The implications for clinical practice remain to be determined, but there can be no doubt that sevoflurane, probably through degradation to compound A, can cause dose-related renal injury. Recognition of this possibility led to a revision of the Warnings section of the package labeling for sevoflurane: "Findings taken from volunteer and patient studies confirmed the potential for renal injury associated with sevoflurane." It adds: "While a level of compound A exposure at which clinical nephrotoxicity might be expected to occur has not been established, it is prudent to consider all of the factors leading to compound A exposure in humans, especially duration of exposure, fresh gas flow rate, and concentration of sevoflurane. During sevoflurane anesthesia the clinician should adjust inspired concentrations and fresh gas flow rate to minimize exposure to compound A." Compound A is also genotoxic (19).

Compound A causes renal injury in rats (8-10,20). However, based on considerations related to the b-lyase pathway and the mechanism of compound A nephrotoxicity, Kharasch et al. questioned whether these results apply to humans (21,22). Our data indicate that the b-lyase pathway does not play an important role in the toxicity of compound A (23,24), and that the discrepancy in our views results from differences in experimental methodology. Specifically, Kharasch et al. test the importance of the b-lyase pathway by injecting compound A intraperitoneally whereas we administer compound A by inhalation. The differences in approach can produce crucial differences in results (25). But the argument is rendered moot by the finding that compound A can injure the human kidney (13).

Desiccated absorbents can break down desflurane, enflurane and isoflurane to produce carbon monoxide (26). Although sevoflurane degradation produces compound A, it does not produce carbon monoxide. The degradation of desflurane, enflurane and isoflurane to carbon monoxide can be prevented by avoiding the use of desiccated absorbents. Prospective clinical studies of carbon monoxide production do not reveal production with desflurane (27), or with isoflurane or enflurane (28), or they reveal minimal production with no difference among anesthetics (29).

Hepatic injury can follow anesthesia with sevoflurane (30-34). For example, a recent study in children suggested that transient increases in alanine aminotransferase (ALT) can occur (35). Transient mild hepatic injury followed sevoflurane anesthesia (but not desflurane anesthesia) in the volunteer study noted above (13), and also occurred in the patients given sevoflurane in the study by Kharasch et al. (16). One case of severe hepatic injury has been reported after anesthesia with desflurane (36).

In summary, desflurane resists biodegradation and degradation by standard carbon dioxide absorbents, whereas sevoflurane degrades and can thereby cause renal injury, especially with prolonged anesthesia at lower inflow rates. Hepatic injury may be more common with sevoflurane than with desflurane. Desiccated absorbents, especially Baralyme, can degrade desflurane to carbon monoxide. Dehydrated Baralyme can increase sevoflurane degradation into compound A (but no carbon monoxide is produced).

REFERENCES

1. Sutton TS, Koblin DD, Gruenke LD, Weiskopf RB, Rampil IJ, Waskell L, Eger EI, II: Fluoride metabolites following prolonged exposure of volunteers and patients to desflurane. Anesth Analg 1991; 73:180-5
2. Holaday DA, Smith FR: Clinical characteristics and biotransformation of sevoflurane in healthy human volunteers. Anesthesiology 1981; 54:100-6
3. Higuchi H, Sumikura H, Sumita S, Arimura S, Takamatsu F, Kanno M, Satoh T: Renal function in patients with high serum fluoride concentrations after prolonged sevoflurane anesthesia. Anesthesiology 1995; 83:449-58
4. Mazze RI, Jamison R: Renal effects of sevoflurane (editorial). Anesthesiology 1995; 83:443-5
5. Goldberg ME, Cantillo J, Larijani GE, Torjman M, Vekeman D, Schieren H: Sevoflurane versus isoflurane for maintenance of anesthesia: are serum inorganic fluoride ion concentrations of concern? Anesth Analg 1996; 82:1268-72
6. Morio M, Fujii K, Satoh N, Imai M, Kawakami U, Mizuno T, Kawai Y, Ogasawara Y, Tamura T, Negishi A, Kumagai Y, Kawai T: Reaction of sevoflurane and its degradation products with soda lime. Toxicity of the by-products. Anesthesiology 1992; 77:1155-64
7. Frink EJ, Jr, Malan TP, Morgan SE, Brown EA, Malcomson M, Brown BR, Jr: Quantification of the degradation products of sevoflurane in two CO2 absorbents during low-flow anesthesia in surgical patients. Anesthesiology 1992; 77:1064-9
8. Gonsowski CT, Laster MJ, Eger EI, II, Ferrell LD, Kerschmann RL: Toxicity of compound A in rats. Effect of increasing duration of administration. Anesthesiology 1994; 80:566-73

9. Gonsowski CT, Laster MJ, Eger EI, II, Ferrell LD, Kerschmann RL: Toxicity of compound A in rats. Effect of a 3-hour administration. Anesthesiology 1994; 80:556-65

10. Keller KA, Callan C, Prokocimer P, Delgado-Herrera L, Friedman MB, Hoffman GM, Wooding WL, Cusick PK, Krasula RW: Inhalation toxicity study of a haloalkene degradant of sevoflurane, compound A (PIFE), in Sprague-Dawley rats. Anesthesiology 1995; 83:1220-32

11. Newton PE, Friedman MB, Hulsebos LH, Rajasekaran D, Walter GL: Acute inhalation toxicity of sevoflurane with 75 or 100 ppm compound A (abstract). The Toxicologist 1998; 42:254

12. Mazze RI: The safety of sevoflurane in humans. Anesthesiology 1992 (editorial); 77:1062-3

13. Eger EI, II, Koblin DD, Bowland T, Balea M, Ionescu P, Laster MJ, Fang Z, Gong D, Sonner J, Weiskopf RB: Nephrotoxicity of sevoflurane vs. desflurane anesthesia in volunteers. Anesth Analg 1997; 84:160-8

14. Eger EI, II, Gong D, Koblin DD, Bowland T, Ionescu P, Laster MJ, Weiskopf RB: Dose-related biochemical markers of renal injury after sevoflurane vs. desflurane anesthesia in volunteers. Anesth Analg 1997; 85:1154-63

15. Bito H, Ikeuchi Y, Ikeda K: Effects of low-flow sevoflurane anesthesia on renal function. Comparison with high-flow sevoflurane anesthesia and low-flow isoflurane anesthesia. Anesthesiology 1997; 86:1231-7

16. Kharasch ED, Frink EJ, Jr, Zagar R, Bowdle TA, Artru A, Nogami WM: Assessment of low-flow sevoflurane and isoflurane effects on renal function using sensitive markers of tubular toxicity. Anesthesiology 1997; 86:1238-53

17. Cantillo J, Goldberg ME, Gratz I, Afsharvand M, Insinga F: Nephrotoxicity of compound A and/or inorganic fluoride ion (F) in normal volunteers. Anesthesiology 1997; 87:A1136

18. Ebert TJ, Frink EJ, Kharasch ED: Absence of biochemical evidence for renal and hepatic dysfunction after 8 hours of 1.25 minimum alveolar concentration sevoflurane anesthesia in volunteers. Anesthesiology 1998; 88:601-10

19. Eger EI, II, Laster MJ, Winegar R, Han C, Gong D: Compound A induces sister chromatid exchanges in Chinese hamster ovary cells. Anesthesiology 1997; 86:918-22

20. Kandel L, Laster MJ, Eger EI, II, Kerschmann RL, Martin J: Nephrotoxicity in rats undergoing a 1-hour exposure to Compound A. Anesth Analg 1995; 81:559-63

21. Kharasch ED, Thorning D, Garton K, Hankins DC, Kilty CG: Role of renal cysteine conjugate b-lyase in the mechanism of compound A nephrotoxicity in rats. Anesthesiology 1997; 86:160-71

22. Jin L, Baillie TA, Davis MR, Kharasch ED: Nephrotoxicity of sevoflurane compound A [fluoromethyl-2,2-difluoro-1-(trifluoromethyl) vinyl ether] in rats: Evidence for glutathione and cysteine

212

      conjugate formation and the role of renal cysteine conjugate b-lyase. Biochem Biophy Res Comm 1995; 210:498-506

23. Martin JL, Laster MJ, Kandel L, Kerschmann RL, Reed GF, Eger EI, II: Metabolism of compound A by renal cysteine-S-conjugate b-lyase is not the mechanism of compound A-induced renal injury in the rat. Anesth Analg 1996; 82:770-4

24. Martin JL, Kandel L, Laster M, Kerschmann RL, Eger EI, II: Studies of the mechanism of the nephrotoxicity of compound A in rats. J Anesth 1997; 11:32-7

25. Eger EI, II, Martin JL: Do the benefits of sevoflurane outweigh the risks? J Anesth 1997; 11:316-7

26. Fang ZX, Eger EI, II, Laster MJ, Chortkoff BS, Kandel L, Ionescu P: Carbon monoxide production from degradation of desflurane, enflurane, isoflurane, halothane, and sevoflurane by soda lime and Baralyme®. Anesth Analg 1995; 80:1187-93

27. Davies MW, Potter FA: Carbon monoxide, soda lime and volatile agents (letter). Anaesthesia 1996; 51:90

28. Baum J, Sachs G, Driesch Cvd, Stanke H-G: Carbon monoxide generation in carbon dioxide absorbents. Anesth Analg 1995; 81:144-6

29. Woehlck HJ, Dunning M, III, Connolly LA: Reduction in the incidence of carbon monoxide exposures in humans undergoing general anesthesia. Anesthesiology 1997; 87:228-34

30. Watanabe K, Hatakenaka S, Ikemune K, Chigyo Y, Kubozono T, Arai T: A case of suspected liver dysfunction induced by sevoflurane anesthesia. Masui 1993; 42:902-5

31. Shichinohe Y, Masuda Y, Takahashi H, Kotaki M, Omote T, Shichinohe M, Namiki A: A case of postoperative hepatic injury after sevoflurane anesthesia. Masui 1992; 41:1802-5

32. Ogawa M, Doi K, Mitsufuji T, Satoh K, Takatori T: Drug induced hepatitis following sevoflurane anesthesia in a child. Masui 1991; 40:1542-5

33. Enokibori M, Miyazaki Y, Hirota K, Sasai S: A case of postoperative fulminant hepatitis after sevoflurane anesthesia. Jap J Anesth 1992; 41:S94

34. Omori H, Seki S, Kanaya N, Imasaki H, Namiki A: A case of postoperative liver damage after isoflurane anesthesia followed by sevoflurane anesthesia. J Jap Soc Clin Anesth 1994; 14:68-71

35. Frink EJ, Jr, Green WB, Jr, Brown EA, Malcomson M, Hammond LC, Valencia FG, Brown BR, Jr: Compound A concentrations during sevoflurane anesthesia in children. Anesthesiology 1996; 84:566-71

36. Martin JL, Plevak DJ, Flannery KD, Charlton M, Poterucha JJ, Humphreys CE, Derfus G, Pohl LR: Hepatotoxicity after desflurane anesthesia. Anesthesiology 1995; 83:1125-9

THE ROLE OF ALPHA$_2$ AGONISTS IN ANESTHESIOLOGY

Mervyn Maze

ADRENERGIC RECEPTORS AND THEIR AGONISTS

The actions of catecholamines are mediated through the activities of agonists on two types of adrenergic receptors, alpha receptors and beta receptors. Alpha receptors are subdivided into two groups, alpha$_1$ (alpha$_{1A}$, alpha$_{1B}$, and alpha$_{1D}$) receptors and alpha$_2$ (alpha$_{2A}$, alpha$_{2B}$, and alpha$_{2C}$) receptors. While alpha receptors were initially divided into subtypes based upon the presynaptic or postsynaptic location of the receptor, this division is no longer reasonable. For example, alpha$_2$ receptors may be located presynaptically, postsynaptically, or extrasynaptically (4). Rather, the various receptor subtypes are best characterized by molecular techniques and cloning. Beta receptors are subdivided into three groups: beta$_1$, beta$_2$, and beta$_3$. These nine different adrenoreceptor subtypes mediate the variety of effects of only two physiologic agonists: epinephrine and norepinephrine.

ALPHA$_1$ ADRENERGIC RECEPTORS

Alpha$_1$ adrenoceptors are present in several tissues including those of the brain, heart, smooth muscle, liver, and spleen (6). Binding of alpha$_1$ agonists at the neuro-effector junction induces a variety of physiologic effects including vasoconstriction, glycogenolysis, and increased heart rate and contractility. The various subtypes, or differences in subtype receptor density in disparate tissues, may modulate the diverse physiologic functions of alpha$_1$ agonists.

213

T. H. Stanley and T. D. Egan (eds.), Anesthesia for the New Millennium, 213–225.

ALPHA 2 ADRENERGIC RECEPTORS

Alpha2 adrenoceptors can be found in the central nervous system (CNS), peripheral nerves (somatic and autonomic), autonomic ganglia, and are ubiquitously distributed throughout the body but especially in tissues innervated by the sympathetic nervous system. Postsynaptic alpha2 adrenoceptors are also found in effector organs such as vascular smooth muscle. Activation of alpha2 receptors produces a variety of responses. Stimulation of presynaptic alpha2 receptors located in the sympathetic nerve endings inhibits the release of the neurotransmitter norepinephrine (4). Activation of postsynaptic receptors by alpha2 agonists in the CNS leads to inhibition of sympathetic activity, decreases in blood pressure and heart rate, decreased arousal, sedation, and relief of anxiety, and binding of agonists to alpha2 adrenoceptors in the spinal cord producing analgesia (4). Peripheral alpha2 receptors in blood vessels mediate vascular smooth muscle contraction (4). Thus, rapid intravenous injection of a potent alpha2 agonist can initially produce an increase in blood pressure resulting from a peripherally induced increased vascular resistance. This effect is transitory, as centrally mediated inhibition of sympathetic activity becomes dominant.

In addition, intestinal motility, salivation, and secretion of gastrointestinal fluids are partially regulated by alpha2 adrenoceptors (4). Activation of alpha2-receptors in the kidneys stimulates sodium and water excretion (4). The physiologic role of alpha2-receptors in the pancreas, adipose tissue, and platelets is incompletely understood. Studies in alpha2-adrenoceptor knockout mice have clarified the role of the various alpha2 receptor subtypes in cardiovascular regulation (7). It appears that the central hypotensive action of alpha2 agonists is due to an action mediated by alpha2A subtype receptors. Increases in systemic vascular resistance and hypertensive responses to alpha2 agonists are a result of stimulation of alpha2B receptors.

BETA ADRENERGIC RECEPTORS

Binding of an agonist to beta-receptor mediates a number of different effects (8). Stimulation of beta1 receptors increases the heart rate, contractility, and cardiac impulse conduction velocity. In addition, beta1 stimulation produces both dilation of renal arterioles and lipolysis. Stimulation of beta2 adrenoceptors produces dilation of arteries in the coronary arterial tree, skeletal muscle, pulmonary vascular bed, kidneys, and systemic veins. Furthermore, binding of beta2 agonists to their receptors results in bronchial smooth muscle relaxation, decreased gastrointestinal motility, and increased secretion of insulin and glucagon. Beta3 adrenoceptors are involved in lipolysis.

EARLY CLINICAL EXPERIENCE WITH ALPHA 2 AGONISTS

Perioperative stress activates a variety of intrinsic defense systems including the sympathetic nervous system, the renin-angiotensin system, and the pituitary-adrenal axis. These changes are accompanied by tachycardia, hypertension, and increased myocardial oxygen utilization. In the presence of hypoxia or coronary heart disease, these alterations can produce myocardial ischemia or necrosis, arrhythmias, and death. As a result, cardiovascular stability is a major concern of intensivists treating critically ill patients. Animal studies on the sympatholytic effects of clonidine, an alpha2 agonist used clinically as an antihypertensive agent, suggested that this drug might improve hemodynamic stability in critically ill patients. As a result, a number of seminal studies were performed to investigate the effects of early alpha2 agonists on cardiovascular responses, vasoactive hormones, and myocardial ischemia in patients undergoing cardiovascular surgery.

Effects of Alpha2 Agonists on the Stress Response

The effects of clonidine on the cardiovascular response to laryngoscopy and tracheal intubation and depth of fentanyl anesthesia were studied in 24 patients undergoing aorto-coronary bypass surgery (9). Patients were hypertensive, had coronary heart disease (New York Heart Association class 3 to 4), and had well-preserved ventricular function. They were divided into two groups of equal size: group 1 received standard premedication (morphine 0.15 mg/kg, intramuscularly and lorazepam 0.03 mg/kg orally); group 2 received the same premedication plus clonidine 5 mcg/kg orally. Depth of anesthesia was monitored with an electroencephalogram (EEG) and fentanyl was administered to shift the

EEG into the delta range in all subjects. No significant differences in hemodynamic measurements were observed in the two groups during the awake period except the stroke volume index, which was significantly greater in the standard therapy group ($P<.05$). In contrast, fentanyl requirements in the clonidine recipients were significantly reduced by 45% compared to standard premedication ($P<.001$). The authors concluded that adequate control of sympathetic-mediated cardiovascular responses was achieved by titrating fentanyl to shift the processed EEG into the delta range. Furthermore, the addition of the alpha2 agonist reduced anesthetic requirements by 45% and decreased the dose of fentanyl to achieve loss of verbal response. Clonidine also shortened the time to achieve ideal intubation conditions and reduced the variability of some of the hemodynamic measurements.

Subsequently, a group of investigators studied the effects of an alpha2-agonist on circulatory dynamics and vasoactive hormones following abdominal aortic grafting (10). After completion of the grafting procedure, 29 patients received a 120-minute intravenous infusion of either placebo or clonidine (7 mcg/kg). Following return to the recovery room, cardiovascular variables were measured and plasma samples were taken for norepinephrine, epinephrine, and vasopressin. Stroke volume was greater ($P<.01$), heart rate was less ($P<.01$), and there were fewer episodes of hypertension ($P<.05$) and tachycardia in the clonidine group. Circulatory interventions were reduced in patients receiving the alpha2 agonist ($P<.05$) and they experienced less shivering. Norepinephrine, epinephrine, and vasopressin concentrations decreased in the clonidine group ($P<.001$, .05, and .05, respectively, versus placebo). The authors concluded that the alpha2 agonist modifies the circulatory and endocrine status after major surgery.

Effects of Alpha2 Agonists on Myocardial Ischemia

Perioperative ischemia is a major healthcare problem. It is the single most important and potentially reversible risk factor for cardiovascular complications and mortality in patients undergoing surgery, whether cardiac or non-cardiac surgery (11). Approximately 30 million Americans undergo non-cardiac surgery annually. Of these, more than 1 million suffer post-surgical cardiovascular morbidity (12). This problem will likely increase in the future as the population ages. As a result, agents that stabilize hemodynamics should decrease ischemia and cardiovascular morbidity and mortality in critically ill patients. In a prospective, randomized, double-blind study, 43 coronary artery bypass graft patients received either clonidine (5 mcg/kg) or placebo in addition to premedication with morphine (0.06 mg/kg) and scopolamine (0.2 mg) (13). Patients treated with the alpha2 agonist had a significantly slower heart rate ($P<.01$), a lower cardiac output ($P<.05$), and transiently higher systemic vascular resistance ($P<.05$) than placebo recipients. Plasma catecholamines were lower in clonidine-treated patients throughout the perioperative procedure with significant differences noted immediately after opening of the chest and following release of the aortic cross-clamp ($P<.05$). Significant ST segment depressions were fewer in patients receiving the alpha2 agonist during the interval between sternotomy and aortic cross-clamping ($P<.01$). Myocardial lactate utilization was significantly increased following cardiopulmonary bypass in patients treated with clonidine. This was particularly prominent at 30 and 60 minutes ($P<.05$). These findings emphasize the myocardial-sparing effect of alpha2 agonists that make them an attractive therapeutic adjuvant in critically ill patients.

Clinical Development of Dexmedetomidine

The results of studies with the early alpha2 agonists suggested that a more selective alpha2 agonist might have significant efficacy as a sedative for critically ill patients in the ICU. Dexmedetomidine is the *d*-enantiomer separated from racemic medetomidine. It is a potent alpha2 adrenoceptor agonist with an alpha2:alpha1 ratio of 1:1620 (14); this is more than sevenfold greater than that of clonidine (Table 2). As of January 1, 1998, a total of 79 studies of the perioperative use of dexmedetomidine has been completed in patients undergoing a variety of types of general and specialized surgery. These studies included assessments of tolerability and pharmacokinetics, dose-response, safety, and efficacy. From these studies, dexmedetomidine has emerged as a drug with several beneficial effects for ICU patients. In contrast to opioids, dexmedetomidine provides its effects of sedation and analgesia without significant respiratory depression. Furthermore, several studies have indicated that the concomitant administration of dexmedetomidine reduces opioid analgesic requirements. The effects seen in the human studies of dexmedetomidine discussed below provided the basis for the formal phase II and III studies of this unique sedative.

SEDATIVE EFFECTS

Sedative effects of dexmedetomidine have been well described. In a comparison of the effects of dexmedetomidine 1.0 mcg/kg and midazolam 0.08 mg/kg, there was a decrease in the amount of thiopentone required for the induction of anesthesia (15). This sedative effect is believed to reflect the action of dexmedetomidine on both presynaptic and postsynaptic alpha2 adrenoceptors in the CNS. Postoperatively, sedation has not been reported to be excessive in patients receiving intravenous dexmedetomidine preoperatively, and some recovery indices (e.g., postoperative mental clouding and nausea, response to verbal commands) appear to have been improved by the drug (16, 17). No differences in postoperative recovery were observed following preoperative intramuscular dexmedetomidine (2.5 mcg/kg) compared to preoperative midazolam premedication (0.08 mg/kg) in patients undergoing abdominal hysterectomy, cholecystectomy, or intraocular cataract surgery (18).

ANXIOLYSIS

Dexmedetomidine appears to have anxiolytic effects. Following intramuscular administration of 2.5 mcg/kg dexmedetomidine, the reduction in anxiety assessed by visual analogue scale was comparable to that observed after intramuscular administration of 0.08 mg/kg midazolam (18) in patients receiving general anesthesia. Administration of 2.4 mcg/kg intramuscular dexmedetomidine as preanesthetic medication in patients prior to gynecologic laparoscopy produced anxiolysis, as assessed by a Profile of Mood States questionnaire (19). Administration of 1.0 mcg/kg intravenous dexmedetomidine 10 minutes prior to exsanguination of the arm also reduced patient apprehension during minor hand surgery under regional anesthesia (20).

ANALGESIC EFFECTS

Perioperative parenteral dexmedetomidine has decreased the requirement for opioids both intraoperatively and postoperatively. For example, the intraoperative requirement for fentanyl during anesthesia was reduced 31% to 56% (18). The analgesic efficacy of dexmedetomidine was assessed during postoperative administration in patients following laparoscopic tubal ligation (21). In a double-blind study of 96 women, patients received either intravenous diclofenac (0.25 mg/kg), oxycodone (60 mcg/kg), or dexmedetomidine (0.2 or 0.4 mcg/kg bolus) until the pain subsided or disappeared. In the group receiving diclofenac, 83% of patients required morphine rescue. In contrast, morphine was required in only 33% of patients receiving either oxycodone or the 0.4 mcg/kg dose of dexmedetomidine.

HEMODYNAMIC EFFECTS

Dexmedetomidine produces hemodynamic stability by effectively blunting both catecholamine and hemodynamic responses to endotracheal intubation (22), surgical stress, emergence from anesthesia, and early recovery (19). In a study of vascular surgical patients with known coronary heart disease or at risk for coronary heart disease, patients received a continuous infusion of either placebo or one of three doses of dexmedetomidine (to achieve target plasma concentrations of 0.15, 0.30, or 0.45 ng/mL) from 1 hour before induction of anesthesia until 48 hours postoperatively. Patients receiving dexmedetomidine had lower preoperative heart rates and systolic blood pressures and had less tachycardia postoperatively compared to placebo recipients. Intraoperatively, however, they required more vasoactive medications to maintain hemodynamics within predetermined limits (23). The results of continuous Holter monitoring suggested a dose-dependent reduction in the severity of postoperative ischemia in patients receiving dexmedetomidine (24). In a study of coronary artery bypass candidates, patients were randomized to receive dexmedetomidine (target plasma concentration, 0.6 ng/mL) or placebo infusion. Compared to the placebo group, patients receiving dexmedetomidine had lower perioperative blood pressures and heart rates on average and required fewer medical interventions to control perioperative hypertension and tachycardia, but required more interventions to control hypotension (25).

ABSENCE OF RESPIRATORY DEPRESSION

Respiratory function was evaluated in a randomized, double-blind comparison of dexmedetomidine (0.2 or 0.4 mcg/kg), oxycodone (60 mcg/kg), or diclofenac (250 mcg/kg) for the treatment of pain following laparoscopic tubal ligation (21). Upon arrival in the recovery room, there were no differences in oxygen saturation or respiratory rate between the study groups. The minimum respiratory frequency was significantly higher in patients receiving 0.4 mcg/kg dexmedetomidine (14 breaths/min) than in patients in the oxycodone group. Administration of oxycodone produced a significantly greater decrease in oxygen saturation than did either the low or high doses of dexmedetomidine. Furthermore, there was no difference in oxygen saturation between the group receiving diclofenac versus dexmedetomidine.

SHIVERING

In the comparative study of dexmedetomidine, oxycodone, and diclofenac as preoperative medication for laparoscopic tubal ligation (21), both dexmedetomidine and oxycodone significantly inhibited postoperative shivering. Postoperative shivering was also reduced in a comparative study of dexmedetomidine (10% incidence) versus midazolam (52% incidence) in patients undergoing elective abdominal hysterectomy (26).

EFFECTS ON PLATELET FUNCTION

Human platelets have receptors for a variety of agonists, including adenosine diphosphate, platelet-activating factor, thrombin, serotonin, epinephrine, and norepinephrine. The adrenergic receptors are predominantly of the alpha$_{2A}$ sub type (27). In view of this association, there has been theoretical concern that administration of an alpha$_2$ agonist might be accompanied by platelet hyperaggregability. Despite this consideration, no evidence of a thrombotic diathesis has been identified in any of the dexmedetomidine clinical trials (28). This lack of clinical manifestations appears to be secondary to a number of factors. While alpha$_2$ agonists can bind to platelet adrenoceptors, experimental evidence suggests that epinephrine per se is not a platelet agonist (at least not in vitro), but instead acts by enhancing the stimulation induced by true agonists (e.g., thrombin, adenosine diphosphate) (29). In addition, any stimulatory activity induced by the agonist activity of dexmedetomidine appears to be counterbalanced by the general sympatholytic activity of the drug. This is supported by experiments on the functional relationships between platelet alpha$_2$ adrenoceptors and general sympathetic activity in hypertensive patients. It appears that platelet alpha$_2$ adrenoceptor density is functionally regulated in parallel with sympathetic nerve activity (30). Consequently, any increased aggregability induced by the agonist is counterbalanced by a reduction in receptor density resulting from the decrease in overall sympathetic tone.

Phase II Results: ICU Sedation

Results of preclinical and early clinical trials demonstrated that dexmedetomidine might have significant efficacy as a sedative in critically ill patients in the ICU. As a result, a Phase II study was conducted to evaluate the efficacy of dexmedetomidine in ICU patients after coronary artery bypass surgery. The study had an open-label limb in which 12 patients received dexmedetomidine and a double-blind limb in which six patients received dexmedetomidine while six received placebo. The goal was to determine how many patients required midazolam (for sedation) or morphine (for analgesia) in addition to dexmedetomidine or placebo to achieve a Ramsay score of 3 or greater. The results are shown in Table 3. No dexmedetomidine recipient in either limb required midazolam, and the number of recipients requiring morphine was also significantly lower than in the placebo group. This study prompted the pivotal Phase III clinical trials.

Phase III Trials

Two phase III dexmedetomidine clinical trials have been conducted. The studies were double-blind, randomized, placebo-controlled, multicenter trials conducted in Canada and Europe. They were designed to evaluate the reduction in requirements for ICU sedation (as measured by administration of other sedative/analgesic agents) in patients receiving dexmedetomidine at comparable levels of sedation, assuming an 80% power calculation. Medication-sparing effects were evaluated for propofol and morphine in one trial and midazolam and morphine in the other

222

trial. Each study was to enroll 420 patients with at least 300 evaluable for efficacy assessment. Patients were to receive either placebo or dexmedetomidine 0.2 to 0.7 mcg/kg/h by continuous infusion, for a maximum duration of 24 hours. Patients were observed and assessed for an additional 24 hours after cessation of the study drug. Case studies from these trials are discussed elsewhere in this monograph.

CONCLUSIONS

Studies with clonidine have shown that an alpha2 agonist can produce hemodynamic stability, reduce the endocrine response to stress, protect against myocardial ischemia, and reduce opioid requirements. These observations led to the development of dexmedetomidine, a novel compound, with more than sevenfold greater alpha2:alpha1 specificity than clonidine. Preclinical, Phase I, and Phase II studies suggest that dexmedetomidine may have significant efficacy when administered as a sedative for critically ill patients in the ICU.

TABLE 1.   PROBLEMS WITH CURRENT SEDATIVE AGENTS

	MIDAZOLAM	PROPOFOL	OPIOIDS
Prolonged weaning	X		X
Respiratory depression	X		X
Severe hypotension	X	X	
Tolerance	X		X
Hyperlipidemia		X	
Increased infection		X	
Constipation			X
Lack of orientation and cooperation	X	X	X*
Abuse potential	X	X	X

*High-dose opioids.

TABLE 2. CLASSIFICATION OF ALPHA ADRENOCEPTORS
IN ORDER OF SELECTIVITY

Agonists		Antagonists	
Alpha$_2$	Dexmedetomidine (1600:1)		Alpha$_2$
	Medetomidine (1620:1)		
	Mivazerol (450:1)		
	Guanabenz*	Atipamezole	
	Guanfacine*	Idazoxan	
	Clonidine* (220:1)	Rauwolcine	
	Xylazine (160:1)	Yohimbine*	
	Dopamine*		
	a-methylnorepinephrine	Tolazoline*	
	Epinephrine*	Phentolamine*	
	Norepinephrine*		
	Phenylephrine*	Corynanthine	
		Phenoxybenzamine*	
Alpha$_1$	Methoxamine*	Prazosin	Alpha$_1$

*Available for clinical use.
Numbers in parentheses indicate alpha$_2$:alpha$_1$ ratio.

REFERENCES

1. Shafer A: Complications of sedation with midazolam in the intensive care unit and a comparison with other sedative regimens. Crit Care Med 1998; 26:947-56.
2. Crippen DW: The role of sedation in the ICU patient with pain and agitation. Crit Care Clin 1990; 6:369-92
3. Shelly MP, Sultan MA, Bodenham A, et al: Midazolam infusions in critically ill patients. Eur J Anaesthesiol 1991; 8:21-7
4. Hayashi Y, Maze M: Alpha$_2$ adrenoceptor agonists and anaesthesia. Br J Anaesth 1993; 71:108-18
5. Tong C, Eisenach JC: a$_2$-Adrenergic agonists. Anesthesiol Clin N Am 1994; 12:49-63
6. Lomasney JW, Cotecchia S, Lefkowitz RJ, et al: Molecular biology of a-adrenergic receptors: implications for receptor classification and for structure-function relationships. Biochem Biophys Acta 1991; 1095:127-39
7. Link RE, Desai K, Hein L, et al: Cardiovascular regulation in mice lacking a$_2$-adrenergic receptor subtypes b and c. Science 1996; 273:803-5
8. Ganong WF: Review of medical physiology. 17th ed. Norwalk, CT: Appleton & Lange; 1995
9. Ghignone M, Quintin L, Duke PC, et al: Effects of clonidine on narcotic requirements and hemodynamic response during induction of fentanyl anesthesia and endotracheal intubation. Anesthesiology 1986; 64:36-42

10. Quintin L, Roudot R, Roux C, et al: Effect of clonidine on the circulation and vasoactive hormones after aortic surgery. Br J Anaesth 1991; 66:108-15

11. Mangano DT, Layug EL, Wallace A, et al: Effect of atenolol on mortality and cardiovascular morbidity after non-cardiac surgery. Multicenter study of perioperative ischemia research group. NEJM 1996; 335:1713-20

12. Mangano DT: Cardiac anesthesia risk management. Multicenter outcome research. JCVA 1994; 8 (suppl 1):10-2

13. Dorman H, Zucker JR, Verrier ED, et al: Clonidine improves perioperative myocardial ischemia, reduces anesthetic requirement, and alters hemodynamic parameters in patients undergoing coronary artery bypass surgery. JCVA 1993; 7:386-95

14. Virtanen R, Savola JM, Saano V, et al: Characterization of the selectivity, specificity and potency of medetomidine as an alpha 2-adrenoceptor agonist. Eur J Pharmacol 1988; 150:9-14

15. Aantaa R, Jaakola ML, Kallio A, et al: A comparison of dexmedetomidine, an alpha2-adrenoceptor agonist, and midazolam as i.m. premedication for minor gynaecological surgery. Br J Anaesth 1991; 67:402-9

16. Aantaa R, Kanto J, Scheinin M, et al: Dexmedetomidine, an alpha2-adrenoceptor agonist, reduces anesthetic requirements for patients undergoing minor gynecological surgery. Anesthesia 1990; 70:407-13

17. Jaakola ML, Ali-Melkkila T, Kanto J, et al: Dexmedetomidine reduces intraocular pressure, intubation responses and anesthetic requirements in patients undergoing ophthalmic surgery. Br J Anaesth 1992; 68:570-5

18. Scheinin H, Jaakola MJ, Sjovall S, et al: Intramuscular dexmedetomidine as premedication for general anesthesia. A comparative multicenter study. Anesthesiology 1993; 78:1065-75

19. Aho M, Scheinin M, Lehtinen AM, et al: Intramuscularly administered dexmedetomidine attenuates hemodynamic and stress hormone responses to gynecologic laparoscopy. Anesth Analg 1992; 75:932-9

20. Jaakola ML: Dexmedetomidine premedication before intravenous regional anesthesia in minor outpatient hand surgery. J Clin Anesth 1994; 6:204-11

21. Aho MS, Erkola OA, Scheinin H, et al: Effect of intravenously administered dexmedetomidine on pain after laparoscopic tubal ligation. Anesth Analg 1991; 73:112-8

22. Scheinin B, Lindgren L, Randell T, et al: Dexmedetomidine attenuates sympathoadrenal responses to tracheal intubation and reduces the need for thiopentone and perioperative fentanyl. Br J Anaesth 1992; 68:126-31

23. Talke P, Li J, Jain U, et al: Effects of perioperative dexmedetomidine infusion in patients undergoing vascular surgery. Anesthesia 1995; 82:620-33

24. Talke P, Mangano DT, Li J, et al: Effect of dexmedetomidine on myocardial ischemia in vascular surgery patient: a safety and dose escalation study. Anesthesiology 1993; 79(3A):A60

25. Heikkila H, Jalonen J, Hynynen M, et al: Dexmedetomidine infusion and perioperative ischaemia in patients undergoing coronary artery bypass surgery. JCVA 1994; 8(suppl 3):54

26. Erkola O, Korttila K, Aho M, et al: Comparison of intramuscular dexmedetomidine and midazolam premedication for elective abdominal hysterectomy. Anesth Analg 1994; 79:646-53

27. Anfossi G, Trovati M: Role of catecholamines in platelet function: pathophysiological and clinical significance. Eur J Clin Invest 1996; 26:353-70

29. Steen VM, Holmsen H, Aarbakke G: The platelet-stimulating effect of adrenaline through alpha-2 adrenergic receptors requires simultaneous activation by a true stimulatory platelet agonist. Evidence that adrenaline per se does not induce human platelet activation in vitro. Thromb Haemost 1993; 70:506-13

30. Noshiro T, Miura Y, Meguro Y, et al: Functional relationships between platelet alpha 2-adrenoceptors and sympathetic nerve activity in clinical hypertensive states. J Hypertens 1990; 8:1097-104

CURRENT CONCEPTS IN ANTI-EMETIC THERAPY

Paul F. White

Nausea, retching and vomiting remain common postoperative complications after ambulatory surgery, irrespective of the anesthetic technique. *Nausea* is defined as a subjectively unpleasant sensation associated with awareness of the urge to vomit. It is usually felt in the back of the throat and epigastrium, occurs in waves and may precede vomiting. *Retching* is defined as labored, spasmodic, rhythmic contractions of the respiratory muscles without the expulsion of gastric contents. *Vomiting or emesis* is the forceful expulsion of gastric contents from the mouth and may alleviate nausea. During vomiting, but not during retching, the hiatal portion of the diaphragm relaxes permitting a transfer of intra-abdominal pressure to the thorax.

The incidence of postoperative nausea and vomiting (PONV) in recent studies has been reported to be in the 20-30% range, which is consistently lower than the 75-80% incidence reported during the "ether" era. Severe (intractable) nausea and vomiting occur in 0.1% (1 in 1000) and is the leading cause of unanticipated admissions after ambulatory surgery (1,2). Although frequently described as a "minor" postoperative complication, it may result in dehydration, electrolyte imbalance, tension on suture lines, venous hypertension, increased bleeding under skin flaps, and delayed discharge (3,4). While nausea and vomiting often occur together, the two conditions should not be considered synonymous. Nausea occurs more frequently than overt vomiting and retching, and can limit patient activity and delay return to work even in the absence of overt retching and vomiting. Thus, PONV may have significant financial implications for the outpatient undergoing a minor elective operation.

T. H. Stanley and T. D. Egan (eds.), Anesthesia for the New Millennium, 227–232.
© *1999 Kluwer Academic Publishers.*

While there have been many investigations of antiemetic drugs for the treatment and/or prevention of PONV in the past, not all have been well controlled, randomized, double-blind studies with an even distribution of confounding factors. A major defect of many otherwise well designed studies is a lack of power analysis to determine the required number of subjects. Consequently, these studies may erroneously conclude that there are no differences between the study groups (type II error). Unfortunately, the wide variability in the definition of nausea and vomiting, the period of postoperative observation, the patient population, and the anesthetic techniques used in previously published studies make it difficult to pool data from multiple studies as part of a meta-analysis. In this lecture, selection of antiemetic drugs and the role of non-pharmacologic techniques will be discussed.

MANAGEMENT OF POSTOPERATIVE NAUSEA AND VOMITING

Despite the many recent advances in ambulatory anesthetic and surgical techniques, postoperative nausea and vomiting remain a "big little problem" (5). PONV is not only distressing to outpatients, it is also a leading cause for delayed discharge and unanticipated hospital admission after ambulatory surgery (6). A recent survey reported that over 35% of outpatients experienced PONV severe enough to delay their resumption of normal activities (7). Interestingly, over half of these patients had not complained of nausea prior to discharge from the ambulatory surgical facility.

It is well accepted that anesthetic agents, the type of surgical procedure, and use of opioid analgesics influence the incidence of PONV. More recently, additional factors that increase the risk of PONV have been identified. These include age, gender, obesity, phase of the menstrual cycle, history of motion sickness or postoperative nausea, pain, anxiety, and hydration status (8,9). While anesthesiologists have little control over many of these factors, some simple measures (e.g., adequate hydration, avoidance of nitrous oxide and reversal agents, limiting the use of opioid analgesics) may be useful in reducing the incidence of PONV (10,11). For example, outpatients hydrated with 20 ml/kg of intravenous fluid had less postoperative morbidity (including nausea) than those receiving only 2 ml/kg (12). The choice of induction agent may also contribute to the reduction of PONV. When propofol was used for induction of anesthesia, there was an 18% decrease in patients experiencing nausea compared to thiopental (13). Propofol administered to induce and maintain anesthesia was even more effective than ondansetron (when given prophylactically to patients receiving a standard thiopental and isoflurane-based anesthetic) in reducing PONV and was associated with fewer requests for rescue antiemetics and a faster early recovery (14).

The prophylactic administration of antiemetics has been shown to be useful in the prevention of PONV in the ambulatory setting. With the introduction of more expensive antiemetic agents (i.e., 5-HT3 receptor antagonists), it is important to consider the efficacy and cost-effectiveness of these newer drugs. Droperidol, 0.625 mg IV, was found to be more cost-effective in preventing PONV than ondansetron, 4 mg IV, in outpatients undergoing gynecologic procedures (15,16). Prophylactic antiemetic therapy is more cost-effective than treatment for operations with a high frequency of emesis. Routine prophylactic use of ondansetron was cost-effective only if the frequency of PONV was greater than 33%, whereas droperidol was cost-effective if the frequency was only 10% (17). The efficacy of prophylactic antiemetics is effected by the timing of their administration. When ondansetron, 4 mg IV, was given at the end of otolaryngologic or gynecologic surgery rather than after induction, it reduced the incidence of PONV and the need for rescue antiemetics (18,19). The beneficial effects of ondansetron in improving recovery were evident in the post-discharge period. Ondansetron has also been successfully used for the treatment of established PONV (20). Ondansetron, 4 mg IV, has been shown to be superior to metoclopramide, 10 mg IV, in the treatment of PONV. However, the use of larger doses (16 mg IV) were no more effective than the smaller dose (21,22).

The use of combinations of antiemetic agents may be more effective than a single agent because of their action at different sites in the chemoreceptor trigger zone. Droperidol, 0.625 mg IV, plus metoclopramide, 10 mg IV, was more effective in preventing postoperative nausea after laparoscopic cholecystectomy than ondansetron, 4 mg IV (23). The use of acupressure and acustimulation at the P6 acupoint has also been investigated but further study is needed to determine the effectiveness of these non-pharmacological techniques (24,25).

SUMMARY

Nausea and vomiting remain the most important anesthetic-related problems following ambulatory surgery (2,3). Although the actual morbidity associated with nausea is relatively low in healthy outpatients, it should not be considered an unavoidable part of the perioperative experience. The availability of an emesis basin for every patient in the PACU is a reflection of our limited success with the available therapeutic modalities. Until recently, there had been little change in the incidence of postoperative emesis following the introduction of halothane into clinical practice. However, the availability of newer anesthetics (e.g., propofol), analgesics (e.g., ketorolac), and muscle relaxants (e.g., mivacurium) appears to have contributed to a recent decline in the incidence of emesis after ambulatory surgery.

REFERENCES

1. Cohen MM, Cameron CB, Duncan PG: Pediatric anesthesia morbidity and mortality in the perioperative period. Anesth Analg 1990; 70:160-7
2. Gold BS, Kitz DS, Lecky JH, Neuhaus JM: Unanticipated admission to the hospital following ambulatory surgery. JAMA 1989;262:3008-10
3. White PF, Shafer A: Nausea and vomiting: causes and prophylaxis. Semin Anesth 1988; 6:300-8
4. Vance JP, Neill RS, Norris W: The incidence and aetiology of postoperative nausea and vomiting in a plastic surgery unit. Br J Plast Surg 1973; 26:336-9
5. Kapur PA: The big "little problem." Anesth Analg 1991;73:243-5
6. Gold BS, Kitz DS, Lecky JH, Neuhaus JM: Unanticipated admission to the hospital following ambulatory surgery. JAMA 1989;262:3008-10
7. Carroll NV, Miederhoff P, Cox FM, Hirsch JD: Postoperative nausea and vomiting after discharge from outpatient surgery centers. Anesth Analg 1995;80:903-9
8. Honkavaara P, Lehtinen AM, Hovorka J, Korttila K: Nausea and vomiting after gynaecological laparoscopy depends upon the phase of the menstrual cycle. Can J Anaesth 1991;38:876-9
9. Beattie WS, Lindblad T, Buckley DN, Forrest JB: The incidence of postoperative nausea and vomiting in women undergoing laparoscopy is influenced by the day of menstrual cycle. Can J Anaesth 1991;38:298-302

10. Divatia JV, Vaidya JS, Badwe RA, Hawaldar RW: Omission of nitrous oxide during anesthesia reduces the incidence of postoperative nausea and vomiting. A meta-analysis. Anesthesiology 1996;85:1055-62

11. Ding Y, Fredman B, White PF: Use of mivacurium during laparoscopic surgery: effect of reversal drugs on postoperative recovery. Anesth Analg 1994;78:450-4

12. Yogendran S, Asokumar B, Cheng DC, Chung F: A prospective randomized double-blinded study of the effect of intravenous fluid therapy on adverse outcomes on outpatient surgery. Anesth Analg 1995;80:682-6

13. Myles PS, Hendrata M, Bennett AM, et al: Postoperative nausea and vomiting. Propofol or thiopentone: does choice of induction agent affect outcome? Anaesth Intensive Care 1996;24:355-9

14. Gan TJ, Ginsberg B, Grant AP, Glass PS: Double-blind, randomized comparison of ondansetron and intraoperative propofol to prevent postoperative nausea and vomiting. Anesthesiology 1996;85:1036-42

15. Tang J, Watcha MF, White PF: A comparison of costs and efficacy of ondansetron and droperidol as prophylactic antiemetic therapy for elective outpatient gynecologic procedures. Anesth Analg 1996;83:304-13

16. Sniadach MS, Alberts MS: A comparison of the prophylactic antiemetic effect of ondansetron and droperidol on patients undergoing gynecologic laparoscopy. Anesth Analg 1997;85:797-800

17. Watcha MF, Smith I: Cost-effectiveness analysis of antiemetic therapy for ambulatory surgery. J Clin Anesth 1994;6:370-7

18. Tang J, Wang BG, White PF, et al: The effect of timing of ondansetron administration on its efficacy, cost-effectiveness, and cost-benefit as a prophylactic antiemetic in the ambulatory setting. Anesth Analg 1998;86:274-82

19. Sun R, Klein KW, White PF: The effect of timing of ondansetron administration in outpatients undergoing otolaryngologic surgery. Anesth Analg 1997;84:331-6

20. Khalil S, Rodarte A, Weldon BC, et al: Intravenous ondansetron in established postoperative emesis in children. S3A-381 Study Group. Anesthesiology 1996;85:270-6

21. Polati E, Verlato G, Finco G, et al: Ondansetron versus metoclopramide in the treatment of postoperative nausea and vomiting. Anesth Analg 1997;85:395-9

22. Rung GW, Claybon L, Hord A, et al: Intravenous ondansetron for post surgical opioid-induced nausea and vomiting. S3A-255 Study Group. Anesth Analg 1997;84:832-8

23. Steinbrook RA, Freiberger D, Gosnell JL, Brooks DC: Prophylactic antiemetics for laparoscopic cholecystectomy: ondansetron versus droperidol plus metoclopramide. Anesth Analg 1996;83:1081-3

24. White PF: Are non pharmacologic techniques useful alternatives to antiemetic drugs for the prevention of nausea and vomiting? Anesth Analg 1997;84:712-4
25. Fan CF, Tanhui E, Joshi S, et al: Acupressure treatment for prevention of postoperative nausea and vomiting. Anesth Analg 1997;84:821-5

NEW INSIGHTS INTO MUSCLE RELAXANTS

Dennis M. Fisher

ONSET: WHICH DRUGS, WHAT TO MONITOR?

Succinylcholine's rapid onset has made it the gold standard for tracheal intubation. In recent years, several new nondepolarizers have become available, their intent being to offer an onset (or duration of action) similar to that of succinylcholine. Published literature offers some insights into this issue but some information is confusing or conflicting. The most important problem is that most studies of muscle relaxants measure onset at the adductor pollicis. Yet, in clinical practice, we are not interested in paralysis of that muscle during onset. Instead, a large dose of muscle relaxant is given to facilitate tracheal intubation and our interest is in the extent of paralysis at the diaphragm and the laryngeal muscles.

Rocuronium, in doses of 600-1200 µg/kg, rapidly produces complete twitch depression. Onset (defined as time to complete depression of adductor pollicis twitch tension) of 600 µg/kg is faster than that of a generous dose of vecuronium, 100 µg/kg (1). Increasing the dose speeds onset. The larger dose, 1200 µg/kg, has an onset nearly identical to that of succinylcholine, limited largely by circulation time (1). Should rocuronium permit tracheal intubation as rapidly as succinylcholine? Intubation studies with rocuronium are few. One study suggested that intubating conditions with rocuronium were excellent at 60 seconds (2). However, this study, like most studies of tracheal intubation, is flawed. In the typical intubation study (3), anesthesia is induced with propofol and an opioid after an opioid premedication. Yet, Scheller et al. (4) demonstrated that propofol (2 mg/kg) plus alfentanil (50-60 µg/kg) without a muscle relaxant produces intubating conditions at 90 seconds comparable to that with a barbiturate and succinylcholine. Thus, all intubation studies

233

T. H. Stanley and T. D. Egan (eds.), Anesthesia for the New Millennium, 233–240.
© 1999 *Kluwer Academic Publishers.*

should be viewed critically to ensure that the anesthetic alone did not ensure adequate success.

If adductor pollicis twitch tension is not a good indicator for the conditions for tracheal intubation and intubation studies are biased by the anesthetic technique, how can one appreciate whether different muscle relaxants will play different roles in facilitating rapid tracheal intubation? Studies by Duvaldestin's group (5) and by Donati and Meistelman (6-8) offer insight into this issue. First, time to peak effect at the adductor pollicis of a subparalyzing dose of vecuronium is 5-6 minutes. In contrast, peak effect at the diaphragm or the laryngeal adductors occurs earlier, at 3-4 minutes and can occasionally exceed peak effect at the adductor pollicis. How can a resistant muscle such as the diaphragm achieve peak effect exceeding that of a sensitive muscle, the adductor pollicis? Studies with vecuronium (9, 10), rocuronium (11), and Organon's new rapid onset nondepolarizer rapacuronium (12) offer an explanation: equilibration between plasma and effect site concentrations is faster for the airway muscles than for the adductor pollicis. This more rapid equilibration presumably results from a greater blood flow (per unit mass) at the airway muscles but might also be explained by differences in drug partitioning in different tissues. The more rapid equilibration results in the airway muscles seeing a more rapid increase in muscle relaxant concentration (fig. 1), thereby permitting a faster time to peak effect and the potential for a greater effect.

If a usual clinical dose of vecuronium produces complete twitch depression in 3-4 minutes, time to complete paralysis at the airway muscles is approximately 2 minutes, the time at which intubation can be accomplished. Rocuronium's onset at the adductor pollicis is more rapid than that of vecuronium; in turn, its onset at the airway muscles is more rapid than at the adductor pollicis (13). Using this principle, it is likely that rocuronium should permit tracheal intubation earlier than vecuronium. The most interesting situation is with mivacurium. The recommended clinical dose — 0.15 mg/kg — produces complete depression at the adductor pollicis at approximately 3 minutes and initial recovery begins at 10-12 minutes. Applying the same principles as for vecuronium and rocuronium, time to maximal depression at the airway muscles should be approximately 2 minutes; in addition, recovery should occur quite early.

This allows only a brief period of maximal paralysis (the "window" for intubation) at the airway muscles (14). If the clinician waits for complete paralysis at the adductor pollicis, then approaches tracheal intubation leisurely, this brief window will have passed and tracheal intubation may not be successful.

The clinical implication of this is obvious — monitoring the adductor pollicis during onset is probably not appropriate because it lags behind the muscles of interest (those of the airway) and will consistently overestimate the time at which intubation can be performed. Two alternate approaches are available — monitor twitch at the orbicularis oculi muscles (6) or monitor the clock. However, during recovery, the adductor pollicis continues to be the conservative measure and remains appropriate.

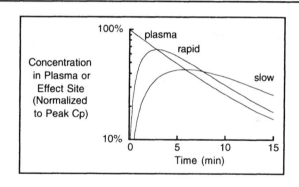

Figure 1. Plasma concentrations and theoretical concentrations at two muscle groups, the adductor pollicis (slow equilibration) and the laryngeal adductors or the diaphragm (rapid equilibration) are shown. All values (shown in %) are normalized to a peak plasma concentration. Concentrations at the airway muscles peak earlier and at a higher value compared to the adductor pollicis, thereby explaining the more rapid onset at the airway muscles and the possibility for greater effect at the "resistant" muscle.

CUMULATION: WHAT   CAUSES   IT?

One important issue regarding muscle relaxants is their predictability with repeated dosing. Pancuronium's duration of action increases markedly with repeated dosing, a phenomenon known as "cumulation." Another manifestation of cumulation is an increased 25%-75% recovery time (the so-called "recovery index") with repeated dosing. In 1986, we explored the etiology of cumulation using pharmacokinetic and pharmacodynamic data for atracurium, vecuronium, and pancuronium (15). We concluded that pancuronium's cumulation resulted from recovery occurring at different points on the plasma concentration (Cp) versus time curve. With small or initial doses, recovery occurred during the steep distribution phase, whereas with larger or repeat doses, recovery occurred during a flatter portion of the Cp curve. The problem here is that pancuronium's decay curve exhibited three distinct phases (three compartments), and the terminal half-life was markedly longer than the distribution half-life. In contrast, the Cp versus time curve for atracurium became log-linear quite rapidly, so that atracurium's recovery was always associated with the same slope of the Cp versus time curve. Vecuronium's Cp versus time curve lay in between and it appeared to be less cumulative than pancuronium but more so than atracurium. That was our perspective in 1986. Was it correct?

We re-examined this issue recently, using a crossover design in volunteers (15). On the first occasion, volunteers received incremental doses of atracurium or vecuronium to determine their individual ED_{95} (16). On the second and third visits, the volunteers received 1.2 or 3.0 times their individual ED_{95} and arterial blood was sampled. The measure of cumulation was the recovery index. Consistent with our simulations, vecuronium's recovery index increased markedly with the larger dose. However, to our surprise, atracurium's recovery index also increased but to a smaller degree than that for vecuronium. We offered three possible explanations for these cumulative effects. First, pharmacokinetics of the muscle relaxants might be nonlinear with dose; however, as anesthesiologists, we would find this unappealing because we depend on linear pharmacokinetics. Second, pharmacodynamics might be non-stationary, i.e., they may change over time. An example of this is phase II block with prolonged administration of succinylcholine. Third, recovery may be shifting from the rapid distribution phase of the Cp versus time curve to a more shallow elimination phase (see above).

The results were surprising. First, the slight cumulation of atracurium could be explained by a shift in the portion of the Cp versus time curve during which recovery occurred. However, a nearly identical shift occurred with vecuronium, yet vecuronium was more cumulative.

This discrepancy can be explained by considering the neuromuscular effects of vecuronium's metabolite, 3-desacetylvecuronium. This metabolite is 80% as potent as vecuronium and has a smaller clearance than vecuronium (17); the metabolite also contributes significantly to the prolonged paralysis observed with prolonged administration of vecuronium in intensive care (18). When concentrations of this metabolite were considered, the greater cumulation of vecuronium compared to atracurium could now be explained, i.e., vecuronium's cumulation with this single small dose results from its metabolite!

Each of the nondepolarizing muscle relaxants is cumulative, although each for different reasons. Mivacurium is slightly cumulative (19). This is probably explained by cumulation of one of mivacurium's stereoisomers (cis-cis), an isomer that comprises only 5% of the administered dose of mivacurium but has an elimination half-life twenty times as long as the other stereoisomers (20). Atracurium's cumulation can be explained by the changing slope of the Cp curve during recovery (contrary to our earlier simulations). Vecuronium's cumulation can be explained by this same phenomenon plus cumulation of its metabolite. Pancuronium's cumulation can probably be explained by the changing slope of the Cp versus time curve. Rocuronium is slightly cumulative (21); as its metabolites are believed to have no neuromuscular effect, cumulation presumably results from a shift of recovery from the steep distribution phase to the flatter elimination phase.

POTENTIATION OF INHALED ANESTHETICS: MORE COMPLICATED THAN WE THOUGHT

Inhaled anesthetics potentiate the effects of muscle relaxants. This potentiation has always been assumed to be beneficial — it permits reduction of the dose of the muscle relaxant, presumably resulting in a smaller concentration of the muscle relaxant at the completion of surgery. In turn, it is assumed that the smaller muscle concentration will permit a more rapid recovery of twitch. This assumption has been challenged in several studies. For example, Baurain et al. (22) administered vecuronium to maintain 90% twitch depression. In one group, isoflurane was discontinued before neostigmine; in a second group, it was continued after antagonism; in the third, no isoflurane was given. The investigators report a number of different measures of recovery; of these, I will focus on tetanic fade 15 minutes after administration of neostigmine. Not surprisingly, the group in which isoflurane was continued had persistent paralysis. In contrast, the group given no isoflurane had minimal residual paralysis. What was most interesting is that the group in which isoflurane had been discontinued (in which end-tidal concentrations were negligible) had persistent paralysis. The investigators speculate, and I agree, that this persistent paralysis in the absence of measurable isoflurane concentrations suggests a persistence of isoflurane (or, at least, its effects) to the neuromuscular junction. The investigators also speculated that recovery from potentiation (which I term "depotentiation") would be better with the newer, less soluble anesthetics.

To examine this issue, we administered vecuronium to volunteers by bolus or by infusion to 85% block during anesthesia with 1.25 MAC of either desflurane or isoflurane (23). In both situations, desflurane potentiated 20% more than isoflurane. Then, while continuing to infuse vecuronium (thereby maintaining constant vecuronium concentrations), we reduced the anesthetic concentration abruptly to 0.75 MAC, then 0.25 MAC. As can be seen in figure 2, the magnitude of recovery (depotentiation) was much greater with desflurane than with isoflurane. This suggests a true advantage to potentiation by desflurane — greater potentiation and greater depotentiation.

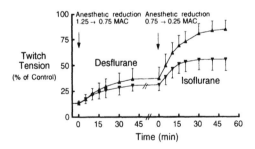

Figure 2. During 1.25 MAC isoflurane or desflurane anesthesia, vecuronium was infused to maintain constant 85% twitch depression. The vecuronium infusion was then continued unchanged while the anesthetic concentration was abruptly decreased to 0.75 MAC, then 0.25 MAC. The magnitude of recovery of twitch tension was markedly greater during the second anesthetic reduction with desflurane compared to isoflurane.

The story of potentiation by inhaled anesthetics is obviously more complicated than we thought — future studies need to examine both potentiation and depotentiation.

REFERENCES

1. Magorian T, Flannery KB, Miller RD: Comparison of rocuronium, succinylcholine, and vecuronium for rapid-sequence induction of anesthesia in adult patients. Anesthesiology 1993; 79: 913-8
2. Wierda JM, de Wit AP, Kuizenga K, Agoston S: Clinical observations on the neuromuscular blocking action of Org 9426, a new steroidal non-depolarizing agent. Br J Anaesth 1990; 64: 521-3
3. Pühringer FK, Khuenl-Brady KS, Koller J, Mitterschiffthaler G: Evaluation of the endotracheal intubating conditions of rocuronium (ORG 9426) and succinylcholine in outpatient surgery. Anesth Analg 1992; 75: 37-40
4. Scheller MS, Zornow MH, Saidman LJ: Tracheal intubation without the use of muscle relaxants: a technique using propofol and varying doses of alfentanil. Anesth Analg 1992; 75: 788-93
5. Chauvin M, Lebrault C, Duvaldestin P: The neuromuscular blocking effect of vecuronium on the human diaphragm. Anesth Analg 1987; 66: 117-22
6. Donati F, Meistelman C, Plaud B: Vecuronium neuromuscular blockade at the diaphragm, the orbicularis oculi, and adductor pollicis muscles. Anesthesiology 1990; 73: 870-5
7. Donati F, Meistelman C, Plaud B: Vecuronium neuromuscular blockade at the adductor muscles of the larynx and adductor pollicis. Anesthesiology 1991; 74: 833-7
8. Donati F, Plaud B, Meistelman C: A method to measure elicited contraction of laryngeal adductor muscles during anesthesia. Anesthesiology 1991; 74: 827-32
9. Bragg P, Fisher DM, Shi J, Donati F, Meistelman C, Lau M, Sheiner LB: Comparison of twitch depression of the adductor pollicis and the respiratory muscles. Pharmacodynamic modeling without plasma concentrations. Anesthesiology 1994; 80: 310-9
10. Fisher DM, Szenohradszky J, Wright PM, Lau M, Brown R, Sharma M: Pharmacodynamic modeling of vecuronium-induced twitch depression. Rapid plasma-effect site equilibration explains faster onset at resistant laryngeal muscles than at the adductor pollicis. Anesthesiology 1997; 86: 558-66
11. Plaud B, Proost JH, Wierda JM, Barre J, Debaene B, Meistelman C: Pharmacokinetics and pharmacodynamics of rocuronium at the vocal cords and the adductor pollicis in humans. Clin Pharmacol Ther 1995; 58: 185-91

12. Wright PMC, Brown R, Lau M, Fisher DM: A pharmacodynamic explanation for the rapid onset/offset of rapacuronium bromide. Submitted to Anesthesiology

13. Wright PM, Caldwell JE, Miller RD: Onset and duration of rocuronium and succinylcholine at the adductor pollicis and laryngeal adductor muscles in anesthetized humans. Anesthesiology 1994; 81: 1110-5

14. Plaud B, Lequeau F, Debaene B, Meistelman C, Donati F: Mivacurium blockade at the adductor muscles of the larynx and adductor pollicis in man. Anesthesiology 1992; 77: A908

15. Wright PMC, Hart P, Lau M, Sharma ML, Gruenke L, Fisher DM: Cumulative characteristics of atracurium and vecuronium. A simultaneous clinical and pharmacokinetic study. Anesthesiology 1994; 81: 59-68

16. Meretoja OA, Wirtavuori K: Two-dose technique to create an individual dose-response curve for atracurium. Anesthesiology 1989; 70: 732-6

17. Caldwell JE, Szenohradszky J, Segredo V, Wright PM, McLoughlin C, Sharma ML, Gruenke LD, Fisher DM, Miller RD: The pharmacodynamics and pharmacokinetics of the metabolite 3-desacetylvecuronium (ORG 7268) and its parent compound, vecuronium, in human volunteers. J Pharmacol Exp Ther 1994; 270: 1216-22

18. Segredo V, Caldwell JE, Matthay MA, Sharma ML, Gruenke LD, Miller RD: Persistent paralysis in critically ill patients after long-term administration of vecuronium. N Engl J Med 1992; 327: 524-8

19. Shanks CA, Fragen RJ, Pemberton D, Katz JA, Risner ME: Mivacurium-induced neuromuscular blockade following single bolus doses and with continuous infusion during either balanced or enflurane anesthesia. Anesthesiology 1989; 71: 362-6

20. Lien CA, Schmith VD, Embree PB, Belmont MR, Wargin WA, Savarese JJ: The pharmacokinetics and pharmacodynamics of the stereoisomers of mivacurium in patients receiving nitrous oxide/opioid/barbiturate anesthesia. Anesthesiology 1994; 80: 1296-302

21. Quill T, Begin M, Glass P, Ginsberg B, Gorback M: Human dose response of ORG 9426 under isoflurane general anesthesia. Anesthesiology 1990; 73: A910

22. Baurain MJ, d'Hollander AA, Melot C, Dernovoi BS, Barvais L: Effects of residual concentrations of isoflurane on the reversal of vecuronium-induced neuromuscular blockade. Anesthesiology 1991; 74: 474-8

23. Wright PM, Hart P, Lau M, Brown R, Sharma ML, Gruenke L, Fisher DM: The magnitude and time course of vecuronium potentiation by desflurane versus isoflurane. Anesthesiology 1995; 82: 404-11

REMIFENTANIL: CLINICAL APPLICATIONS

Talmage D. Egan

INTRODUCTION

Remifentanil is a new congener of the fentanyl family of opioids that was approved for use as a supplement to general anesthesia by the United States Food and Drug Administration in 1996 (1). Remifentanil is now available in numerous countries internationally, but it is still in the early stages of clinical application and development (2).

Pharmacodynamically, remifentanil is in most regards indistinguishable from the other fentanyl congeners, producing analgesia, respiratory depression and other effects typical of the fentanyl derivatives. Remifentanil's unique feature is its short-acting pharmacokinetic profile. Remifentanil's ester structure renders it susceptible to widespread ester hydrolysis, resulting in very rapid metabolism. Remifentanil thus constitutes the first true *"ultra*short acting" opioid.

The aim of this review is to describe briefly remifentanil's clinical pharmacology and to discuss its clinical application.

PHYSICOCHEMICAL PROPERTIES

Remifentanil is related to the phenylperperidine compounds. Known in its early development as GI87084B, it is the hydrochloride salt of 3-[4-methoxycarbonyl-4-[(1-oxopropyl)phenylamino]-1–piperidine] propanoic acid methyl ester.

Remifentanil's physicochemical properties have important implications for clinical use (2,3). Like the other fentanyl congeners,

Author's Note: This chapter was adapted with permission from Egan TD: The clinical pharmacology of remifentanil: a brief review.   J Anesth 1998;12:195-204.

T. H. Stanley and T. D. Egan (eds.), Anesthesia for the New Millennium, 241–261.
© 1999 *Kluwer Academic Publishers.*

remifentanil is a weak base that is quite lipid soluble (octanol/water partition coefficient of 19.9 at pH 7.4). With a pKa of 7.1, it exists mostly in the unionized form at physiologic pH. It is highly bound (70-80%) to plasma proteins, mostly alpha-1-acid glycoprotein. Some of remifentanil's physicochemical properties are listed in table 1.

Despite the fact that remifentanil is highly protein bound, remifentanil's comparatively low pKa means that the diffusible fraction (the unbound, unionized portion) is high. A high diffusible fraction, in combination with moderate lipid solubility, makes remifentanil a rapid onset opioid.

Remifentanil free base is formulated with glycine. Because glycine is an important inhibitory neurotransmitter in the central nervous system of mammals, in addition to typical opioid effects, remifentanil causes a reversible motor weakness when administered intrathecally in rodents (4,5). Thus, remifentanil is not approved for intrathecal or epidural use.

Table 1. Representative remifentanil physicochemical properties and pharmacokinetic parameters

pKa	7.1
% un-ionized at pH 7.4	67
Octanol/H_2O partition coefficient	17.9
% bound to plasma protein	80?
Diffusible fraction (%)	13.3?
t 1/2 alpha, min	.5-1.5
t 1/2 beta, min	5-8
t 1/2 gamma, h	0.7-1.2
Vdc, L/kg	.06-.08
Vdss, L/kg	0.2-0.3
Clearance ml/min/kg	30-40

Abbreviations: t 1/2 alpha, first distribution half-life; t 1/2 beta, second distribution half-life; t 1/2 gamma, elimination half-life; Vdc, volume of distribution of central compartment; Vdss, volume of distribution at steady state; ? indicates not yet well known.

Remifentanil is supplied as a white powder that readily dissolves in water, normal saline or lactated ringers solution (or these same solutions containing dextrose). Because remifentanil is not stable in solution for long periods of time, it must be reconstituted within 24 hours prior to use.

Two methods are now available for the measurement of remifentanil in whole blood. Although they employ different methodologies, they have similar quantitation limits and ranges (6,7).

METABOLISM

Remifentanil undergoes widespread extrahepatic hydrolysis by non-specific esterases in blood and tissue. Incubation of remifentanil in fresh human whole blood demonstrates that remifentanil can undergo ester cleavage *in vitro*, suggesting that the same metabolic pathway is operative *in vivo* (9).

The primary metabolic pathway for remifentanil is de-esterification to form a carboxylic acid metabolite, GI90291. About 90% of the drug is recovered in the urine in the form of this acid metabolite (10). GI90291 is excreted unchanged in the urine and is therefore dependent on renal clearance mechanisms (see Special Populations).

Remifentanil's metabolic pathway is shown in figure 1. While most remifentanil hydrolysis probably occurs in tissue (perhaps because it is distributed so quickly), the site of remifentanil metabolism within the vasculature appears to be inside the red cell (11).

The body's capacity to metabolize esters like remifentanil is very substantial and does not appear to be influenced by coadministration of drugs that are metabolized by the same enzyme systems such as esmolol (12). However, whether this applies to other commonly used esters such as succinylcholine remains to be demonstrated.

PHARMACODYNAMICS

Remifentanil is a pure mu receptor agonist whose opioid receptor activity has been demonstrated *in vitro*. Remifentanil inhibits electrically evoked contraction in guinea-pig ileum and rat and mouse vas deferens, three isolated animal tissues commonly used to demonstrate opioid receptor activity (13). In these studies remifentanil exhibited its effect at the mu-subtype of opioid receptor, as evidenced by the complete reversibility of the effects by naloxone. Naloxone antagonism of remifentanil's effects has also been demonstrated in humans (14).

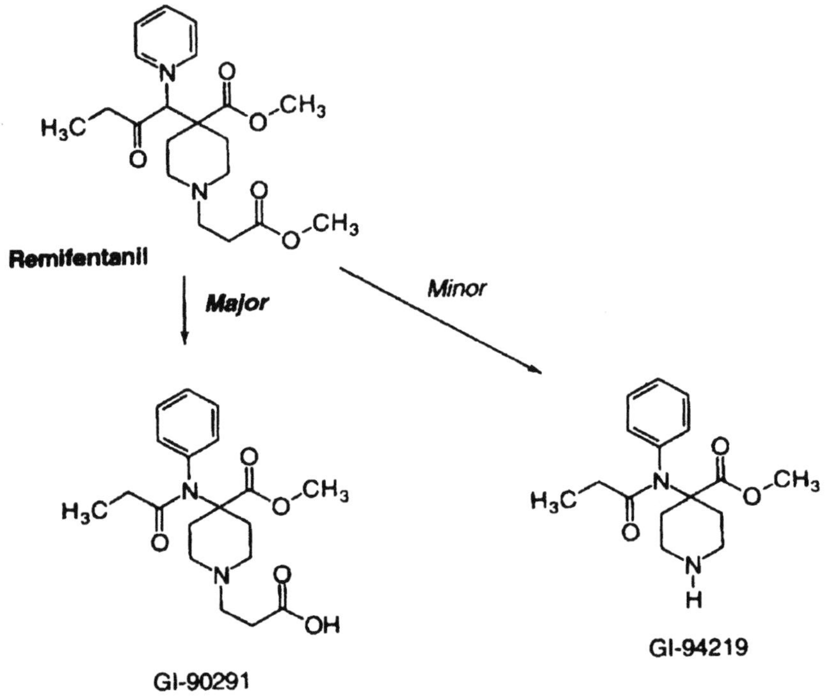

Figure 1. Remifentanil's metabolic pathway. De-esterification by nonspecific plasma and tissue esterases to form a carboxylic acid metabolite (GI90291) is the primary metabolic pathway. N-dealkylation of remifentanil to GI94219 is a minor metabolic pathway (From Egan [2], with permission).

As a pure mu-agonist, remifentanil produces all the opioid effects characteristic of the fentanyl family of opioids. Its therapeutic effects therefore include dose-related analgesia and sedation.

Remifentanil's effects on the central nervous system are reflected in the raw electroencephalograph (EEG). At high doses, remifentanil produces a slowing in frequency and an increase in amplitude that translate into a decrease in the spectral edge parameter (15). These changes are regarded as the EEG fingerprint of this drug class (16). Figure 2 illustrates the typical spectral edge changes observed when human volunteers receive a brief but high-dose infusion of remifentanil.

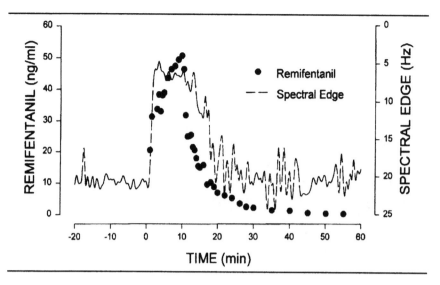

Figure 2. Representative changes in remifentanil blood concentrations and the EEG spectral edge parameter produced by a 10 minute infusion of remifentanil at 3 mcg/kg/min. Note the very close relationship between changes in blood concentration and changes in the spectral edge with a rapid return of the spectral edge to baseline values as the remifentanil concentration declines (from Egan et al [15], with permission).

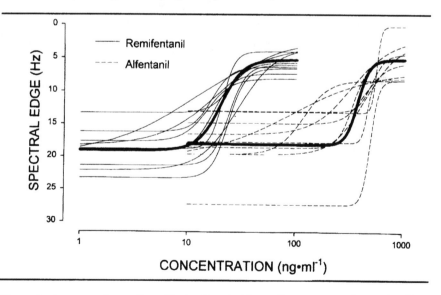

Figure 3. A comparison of remifentanil and alfentanil potency as determined by the EEG. Ten adult males received infusions of remifentanil and alfentanil on separate occasions at dosages sufficient to produce maximal changes on the EEG. Each curve represents the concentration-effect relationship of a single volunteer. The bold curves represent the mean concentration-effect relationship for each drug. As measured by the EEG, remifentanil is about 20-30 times more potent than alfentanil (From Egan et al [15], with permission).

In terms of potency, remifentanil is substantially more potent than alfentanil and slightly less potent than fentanyl. These potency estimates have been made using MAC (minimum alveolar concentration) reduction and EEG methods (15,17-19). Figure 3 contrasts the potency of remifentanil compared to alfentanil using the EEG as the measure of drug effect.

Remifentanil's adverse effect profile is also essentially indistinguishable from the previously marketed fentanyl congeners. Most importantly, remifentanil produces a dose-dependent increase in the partial pressure of carbon dioxide as a result of ventilatory depression. Remifentanil's respiratory depression closely parallels remifentanil blood concentrations and has thus been exploited as a measure of drug effect for pharmacodynamic modeling purposes (20).

The hemodynamic effects of remifentanil are also characteristic of the fentanyl series of opioids. Remifentanil causes dose-dependent decreases in heart rate, arterial blood pressure and cardiac output (21). At high doses, severe bradycardia has been reported secondary to remifentanil (22). These cardiovascular effects are thought to be at least in part related to a centrally mediated increase in vagal tone (23). Unlike morphine, the decrease in arterial blood pressure observed with remifentanil is not secondary to histamine release (24).

Other side effects that are expected with mu-agonists have also been reported in association with remifentanil. These adverse effects include nausea, vomiting, pruritus and muscle rigidity (2). Intraoperative awareness has also been reported in association with remifentanil (25).

PHARMACOKINETICS

Remifentanil's short acting pharmacokinetic profile is its unique pharmacologic feature. In terms of the rapidity with which concentrations fall after stopping an infusion, remifentanil is dramatically different from the other fentanyl congeners.

Remifentanil's pharmacokinetics are best described by a three compartment model (15,17,26,27). Its clearance is several times greater than hepatic blood flow which is consistent with widespread extrahepatic metabolism (28). As with the other fentanyl congeners, remifentanil is widely distributed in body tissues with a steady-state distribution volume of approximately 20-40 liters (15,17,26,27). Unlike the other fentanyl congeners, remifentanil is not sequestered or taken up by the lung to any substantial degree (29).

Numerous "high resolution" studies have confirmed remifentanil's short-acting pharmacokinetic profile (15,17,26,27). Table 1 lists some parameters that are representative of remifentanil's pharmacokinetics (17).

A graphic representation of remifentanil's context sensitive half-time ($CST_{1/2}$) is perhaps the most clinically meaningful way of representing remifentanil's pharmacokinetics. Defined as the time required to achieve a 50% decrease in concentration after stopping an infusion targeted to steady-state, the $CST_{1/2}$ is a useful means of contrasting the clinical implications of multicompartment pharmacokinetic parameters (30,31). Figure 4 illustrates the $CST_{1/2}$ of remifentanil compared to the other members of the fentanyl series of opioids. Remifentanil's $CST_{1/2}$ is short (approximately 3-4 minutes) and is independent of infusion duration (15,17,26,27). The robustness of remifentanil's $CST_{1/2}$ has been confirmed prospectively (20). Thus, remifentanil can be viewed as a truly rapid offset opioid.

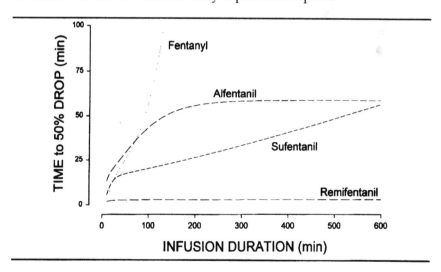

Figure 4. A graphical representation of the context sensitive half-times ($CST_{1/2}$) for remifentanil and the other fentanyl congeners using pharmacokinetic parameters from the literature. The $CST_{1/2}$ simulates the time required for a 50% decrease in plasma concentration after termination of a continuous infusion targeted to a steady-state level. Note the short, time-independent $CST_{1/2}$ of remifentanil (From Egan et al [26], with permission).

Remifentanil's latency-to-peak effect is also rapid and is comparable with that of alfentanil. Remifentanil's $t_1/2_{ke0}$, the parameter used to characterize the delay between peak drug levels in the plasma (or blood) and peak drug effect, is similar to that of alfentanil as reported in several human volunteer studies, some using the EEG and others using an experimental pain method (10,15,17). Figure 5 depicts the time required to reach peak effect-site concentration (and therefore peak effect) after bolus administration of the fentanyl congeners. Like alfentanil, remifentanil reaches peak effect-site concentration within 1-2 minutes after bolus injection and then begins to decline (32). This means that remifentanil can be regarded as a rapid onset agent.

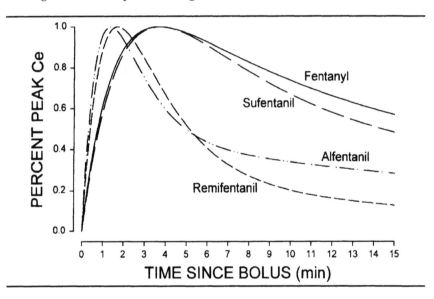

Figure 5. A computer simulation of the time required to reach peak effect site concentration after bolus administration of fentanyl, alfentanil, sufentanil and remifentanil using pharmacokinetic parameters from the literature. This is a graphic illustration of the plasma-biophase equilibration process for these drugs. Ce is the effect site concentration; a bolus injection was made at time 0. (From Egan et al [32], with permission).

SPECIAL POPULATIONS

Age

Advancing age has an important influence on remifentanil pharmacokinetics and pharmacodynamics (17). Remifentanil clearance and central distribution volume decline with age. Similarly, the EC_{50}, the concentration necessary for 50% of maximal effect as measured by the EEG, also declines substantially with age. This means that remifentanil is significantly more potent in the elderly and that it is not cleared as quickly (the blood and effect-site also equilibrate more slowly). These age-related changes translate into a 50-70% dosage reduction in the elderly (i.e., patients over approximately 60 years) (33). Figure 6 illustrates the change in potency as a patient ages.

Comparatively little is known about remifentanil in the pediatric population. However, the available data indicate that remifentanil is also a short acting drug in children and newborns (34,35).

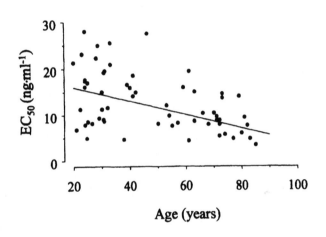

Figure 6. The relationship of age and remifentanil potency as measured by the EEG. Like the other fentanyl congeners, as age increases the concentration required to achieve 50% of maximal brain depression (i.e., the EC_{50}) on the EEG decreases (From Minto et al [17], with permission).

Weight

Body weight is another important factor in the formulation of remifentanil dosage regimens. Remifentanil pharmacokinetic parameters are more closely related to lean body mass than to total body weight (36). In other words, patients who weigh more do not necessarily have a proportional increase in metabolic capacity. This is consistent with the observation that over 90% of metabolic processes are thought to occur in lean tissue (37).

This means that obese patients, particularly morbidly obese patients, do not need to receive a higher dose (i.e., a weight normalized dose).

Remifentanil dosages should be calculated based on lean body mass or ideal body weight and not total body weight. Truly obese patients who receive a total body weight based dosage are more likely to suffer bradycardia, hypotension and other adverse effects (36).

Gender

Gender does not appear to have an important influence on remifentanil pharmacokinetics or pharmacodynamics. In a large, high resolution study, Minto showed that neither the pharmacokinetic nor the pharmacodynamic parameters significantly changed with gender. Remifentanil dosage regimens can therefore be formulated irrespective of patient gender.

Kidney Function

Remifentanil pharmacokinetics are not influenced by renal function. The pharmacokinetics of remifentanil administered by infusion for four hours to renal dialysis patients have been compared to control subjects (38). Remifentanil pharmacokinetics in renal impairment are not appreciably different from normal subjects.

Because it is cleared by the kidney, concerns have been raised regarding the fate of the metabolite, GI90291, in renal failure (2,39). With a potency that is several orders of magnitude less than the parent compound, current evidence suggests that even though GI90291 may rise to levels that are 25 times those of remifentanil in the face of renal failure, it is unlikely to exert any pharmacodynamic activity (38).

Hepatic Failure

Like renal failure, hepatic failure does not appear to alter remifentanil pharmacokinetics. The pharmacokinetic behavior of remifentanil in patients awaiting liver transplantation for end-stage hepatic disease has been investigated (40). Remifentanil pharmacokinetics were unchanged by severe liver disease at doses up to 0.25 mcg/kg/min. The findings of this study are bolstered by the observation that remifentanil clearance continues unchanged during the anhepatic phase of orthotopic liver transplantation (41). Interestingly, patients with end-stage liver disease may be pharmacodynamically more sensitive to remifentanil (40).

PHARMACOGENETICS

Because of remifentanil's esterase dependent metabolic pathway, questions regarding remifentanil metabolism in pseudocholinesterase deficiency patients inevitably arise. *In vitro* tests indicate that remifentanil is not a good substrate for butylcholinesterase (i.e., pseudocholinesterase) (11), suggesting that no dosage reduction will be necessary in patients with any subtype of pseudocholinesterase deficiency. When remifentanil is introduced *in vitro* into plasma harvested from pseudocholinesterase deficient volunteers, its rate of metabolism is not different from that observed in the plasma of normal controls (42).

CLINICAL APPLICATIONS

Although it is still too early to predict with confidence what clinical niche remifentanil will ultimately occupy, remifentanil is obviously best suited for cases where its responsive pharmacokinetic profile can be exploited. Remifentanil is perhaps best applied to cases when rapid recovery is desirable, when the anesthetic requirement rapidly fluctuates, when opioid titration is unpredictable or difficult, when there is a substantial danger to opioid overdose, or when a "high dose" opioid technique is advantageous but the patient is not going to be mechanically ventilated postoperatively.

In this context, one very unique aspect of remifentanil is that its use mandates a change in the traditional pharmacologic ratios of "balanced anesthesia" (46). Because it is so pharmacokinetically evanescent, remifentanil can be infused to a profound level of opioid effect and yet enable the return of spontaneous ventilation only a few minutes later. This means that it is possible to do a "high dose" opioid technique such as is commonly used for cardiac anesthesia (for any kind of case) without committing a patient to mechanical ventilation postoperatively.

In very practical terms, the clinician must answer a few simple questions in deciding whether remifentanil might be appropriate for any given case: Is rapid recovery absolutely essential (e.g., neuroanesthesia, outpatient procedures)? Is the control of autonomic responses to noxious stimuli important and perhaps problematic with longer acting opioids (e.g., patient with severe coronary artery disease for a brief outpatient procedure)? Will determination of the proper opioid dosage be difficult (e.g., children, elderly, hepatic disease patient)? Is there a substantial danger to opioid overdose (e.g., during fiberoptic intubation of the difficult airway)? When the answers to these questions are yes, remifentanil may be helpful.

General Anesthesia

Remifentanil can be infused as a supplement to general anesthesia in combination with either inhaled vapor or intravenous sedative hypnotics such as propofol. It has been used successfully for both inpatient and outpatient general anesthesia (47-49).

Interestingly, remifentanil in combination with propofol for anesthetic induction can reportedly produce adequate conditions for tracheal intubation without muscle relaxants (50). Remifentanil at low doses has also been successfully used as a supplement to inhaled anesthetic without muscle relaxants in patients spontaneously ventilating through a laryngeal mask airway for outpatient surgery (51). Remifentanil, like the other opioids, should not be regarded as a complete anesthetic. It is not suitable as a sole induction or maintenance agent (52).

Conscious Sedation-Analgesia

Remifentanil is also approved by the United States Food and Drug Administration as the analgesic component of conscious sedation during monitored anesthesia care. It can be infused in combination with propofol (by infusion) or midazolam (by bolus dosing) to provide relief of anxiety and pain during procedures where local anesthesia is infiltrated at the site of the operation (or for procedures where no local anesthesia is necessary). It can also be infused as an adjunct to procedures performed under regional block (53).

For practical purposes, remifentanil should not be viewed as an appropriate single agent for monitored anesthesia care when significant sedation is desired. It is difficult to produce substantial sedation with remifentanil alone without producing significant respiratory depression. Although remifentanil can be used alone, optimal conscious sedation and analgesia are more easily achieved with remifentanil in combination with a sedative-hypnotic such as propofol or midazolam (54, 55).

Neuroanesthesia

Rapid emergence from anesthesia is a priority after neurosurgical procedures so that a neurologic assessment can take place before leaving the operating room. Remifentanil's short acting pharmacokinetic profile can be exploited to promote a quick return of consciousness after neurosurgical procedures to allow for a neurological exam shortly after the surgeons have finished their work.

Remifentanil's effects on cerebral physiology appear to be similar to the other fentanyl congeners, although they are shorter-lived (56). When ventilation is controlled, remifentanil does not cause an increase in intracranial pressure when infused to patients undergoing craniotomy (57).

Remifentanil has been used successfully as an alternative to fentanyl as part of a balanced anesthetic technique for resection of supratentorial lesions. In a series of 63 adult craniotomy patients who were randomized to receive either remifentanil or fentanyl, remifentanil was thought to help promote a rapid emergence that did not require the administration of naloxone (58). Remifentanil in combination with propofol has also been reported to provide excellent conditions for awake craniotomy (59).

Cardiac Anesthesia

Comparatively little is known about remifentanil's pharmacokinetics during cardiopulmonary bypass (CPB). For example, how much remifentanil is sequestered by the CPB circuit is unknown. It is clear, however, that remifentanil remains a very short-acting drug despite CPB (29). During the hypothermic portion of CPB remifentanil's clearance decreases by about 20% and then returns to prebypass levels after rewarming (60).

Remifentanil has been used successfully as a means of promoting "fast-track" anesthesia (i.e., early extubation of the trachea) after cardiopulmonary bypass operations (61). While the preliminary indications have been promising, the results of ongoing work in this area will be required to establish the utility of remifentanil for cardiac anesthesia.

Pediatric Anesthesia

Compared to the adult population, relatively little information is available regarding remifentanil's clinical pharmacology and clinical use in pediatric patients. As noted earlier, it appears that remifentanil's pharmacokinetics are not markedly different in children (including neonates) compared to adults. Because it can be difficult to determine how much opioid will provide the analgesic component of anesthesia without preventing the return of spontaneous ventilation at the end of a pediatric procedure, some have suggested that remifentanil may be the ideal opioid for use in pediatric anesthesia (62).

Obstetric Anesthesia

As might be expected for a recently approved drug, there is very little information available about remifentanil in obstetric anesthesia. Only one study has documented the apparent safety of intravenous remifentanil infusion during cesarean section under epidural anesthesia (63). The data from this study suggest that remifentanil readily crosses the placenta with an umbilical vein to maternal artery ratio of 0.88. This study also indicates that remifentanil probably has a short duration of action in the neonate whose mother received the drug just before delivery because the umbilical artery to umbilical vein ratio was only 0.29, suggesting that the fetus is metabolizing (or distributing) the drug rapidly. Another report proposes that remifentanil may be useful by infusion as an adjunctive analgesic for labor pain such as before or during epidural catheter placement (64).

It is important to emphasize that remifentanil is not approved for obstetric anesthesia by the United States Food and Drug Administration. The effect of remifentanil on uterine blood flow and contractility is unknown. Whether or not neonates whose mothers received remifentanil in substantial doses just prior to delivery would be adversely affected by remifentanil is also relatively unexplored. These and other issues may require full examination before widespread use of remifentanil in parturients can be advocated.

Acute Pain Management

Remifentanil is also approved for the treatment of acute postoperative pain in the post anesthesia care unit and the intensive care unit. Several studies have demonstrated the efficacy of remifentanil for this indication. With a remifentanil infusion ongoing in the recovery room at rates ranging from about 0.05 to 0.1 mcg/kg/min, a high proportion of patients rate their pain as either mild or absent after major surgery (65, 66).

Making the transition from remifentanil intraoperatively to a longer-acting analgesic postoperatively is one of the challenging aspects of using remifentanil. Because remifentanil is metabolized so rapidly, there is the possibility of a rapid decline in analgesia during emergence from anesthesia unless an analgesic infusion of remifentanil is maintained or unless the transition to another longer-acting analgesic is made prior to emergence (2, 65). Anesthesiologists are accustomed to switching from the intraoperative opioid (usually one of the fentanyl congeners) to the postoperative opioid (usually morphine or meperidine) in the post anesthesia care unit. With remifentanil, it is necessary to make this transition before the end of anesthesia (e.g., 100 mcg of fentanyl about 15 minutes before the end of the operation or 5-10 mg of morphine about 30 minutes before the end of the operation).

Future Applications

In the future, remifentanil may be used for a host of other applications, including some outside the operating room. For example, remifentanil may be useful by bolus injection to provide analgesia during short, painful diagnostic or therapeutic procedures such as lumbar puncture, central venous catheterization or wound dressing changes. It may also be useful by continuous infusion in the intensive care unit for the conscious sedation-analgesia of mechanically ventilated patients. In the chronic pain arena, remifentanil may be useful as a diagnostic tool in the ambulatory clinic in determining whether a patient with a complex chronic pain syndrome is or is not responsive to opioid analgesics. These and other potential applications for remifentanil are currently under study.

SUMMARY

Because it is still in its clinical infancy, it is difficult to predict with confidence exactly what role remifentanil will ultimately play in the delivery of anesthesia (and in other settings). It is clear, however, that remifentanil is a new pharmacologic tool that has exciting potential that was not possible with the longer-acting opioids. Based on its familiar, fentanyl-like pharmacodynamic behavior and its short-acting pharmacokinetic profile, remifentanil may well be advantageous in a variety of settings in which profound opioid effect with subsequent rapid return of spontaneous ventilation and consciousness is desirable. Ongoing research and widespread clinical use will be required before the theoretical advantages associated with a short-acting opioid can be fully explored and confirmed.

REFERENCES

1. Anonymous (1996) Remifentanil approved for anesthesia use [news]. Am J Health Syst Pharm 53:1079-2082
2. Egan TD (1995) Remifentanil pharmacokinetics and pharmacodynamics. A preliminary appraisal. Clin Pharmacokinet 29:80-94
3. Glass PS (1995) Remifentanil: a new opioid. J Clin Anesth 7:558-63
4. Buerkle H, Yaksh TL (1996) Continuous intrathecal administration of shortlasting mu opioids remifentanil and alfentanil in the rat. Anesthesiology 84:926-35
5. Buerkle H, Yaksh TL (1996) Comparison of the spinal actions of the mu-opioid remifentanil with alfentanil and morphine in the rat. Anesthesiology 84:94-102
6. Grosse CM, Davis IM, Arrendale RF, Jersey J, Amin J (1994) Determination of remifentanil in human blood by liquid-liquid extraction and capillary GC-HRMS-SIM using a deuterated internal standard. J Pharm Biomed Anal 12:195-203
7. Selinger K, Lanzo C, Sekut A (1994) Determination of remifentanil in human and dog blood by HPLC with UV detection. J Pharm Biomed Anal 12:243-8
8. Haidar SH, Liang Z, Selinger K, Hamlett L, Eddington ND (1996) Determination of remifentanil, an ultra-short-acting opioid anesthetic, in rat blood by high performance liquid chromatography with ultraviolet detection. J Pharm Biomed Anal 14:1727-32
9. Feldman PL, James MK, Brackeen MF, Bilotta JM, Schuster SV, Lahey AP, Lutz MW, Johnson MR, Leighton HJ (1991) Design, synthesis, and pharmacological evaluation of ultrashort- to long-acting opioid analgetics. J Med Chem 34:2202-8
10. Glass PS, Hardman D, Kamiyama Y, Quill TJ, Marton G, Donn KH, Grosse CM, Hermann D (1993) Preliminary pharmacokinetics and pharmacodynamics of an ultra-short-acting opioid: remifentanil (GI87084B). Anesth Analg 77:1031-40

257

11. Selinger K, Nation RL, Smith A (1995) Enzymatic and chemical hydrolysis of remifentanil. Anesthesiology 83:A385
12. Haidar SH, Moreton JE, Liang Z, Hoke JF, Muir KT, Eddington ND (1997) Evaluating a possible pharmacokinetic interaction between remifentanil and esmolol in the rat. J Pharm Sci 86:1278-82
13. James MK, Feldman PL, Schuster SV, Bilotta JM, Brackeen MF, Leighton HJ (1991) Opioid receptor activity of GI 87084B, a novel ultra-short acting analgesic, in isolated tissues. J Pharmacol Exp Ther 259:712-8
14. Amin HM, Sopchak AM, Esposito BF, Henson LG, Batenhorst RL, Fox AW, Camporesi EM (1995) Naloxone-induced and spontaneous reversal of depressed ventilatory responses to hypoxia during and after continuous infusion of remifentanil or alfentanil. J Pharmacol Exp Ther 274:34-9
15. Egan TD, Minto CF, Hermann DJ, Barr J, Muir KT, Shafer SL (1996) Remifentanil versus alfentanil: comparative pharmacokinetics and pharmacodynamics in healthy adult male volunteers. Anesthesiology 84:821-33
16. Egan TD, Muir KT, Stanski DR, Shafer SL (1996) The EEG versus clinical measures of opioid potency: defining the EEG-clinical potency fingerprint with application to remifentanil. Anesthesiology 85:A349
17. Minto CF, Schnider TW, Egan TD, Youngs E, Lemmens HJ, Gambus PL, Billard V, Hoke JF, Moore KH, Hermann DJ, Muir KT, Mandema JW, Shafer SL (1997) Influence of age and gender on the pharmacokinetics and pharmacodynamics of remifentanil. I. Model development. Anesthesiology 86:10-23
18. Michelsen LG, Salmenpera M, Hug CC, Jr., Szlam F, VanderMeer D (1996) Anesthetic potency of remifentanil in dogs. Anesthesiology 84:865-72
19. Lang E, Kapila A, Shlugman D, Hoke JF, Sebel PS, Glass PS (1996) Reduction of isoflurane minimal alveolar concentration by remifentanil. Anesthesiology 85:721-8
20. Kapila A, Glass PS, Jacobs JR, Muir KT, Hermann DJ, Shiraishi M, Howell S, Smith RL (1995) Measured context-sensitive half-times of remifentanil and alfentanil [see comments]. Anesthesiology 83:968-75
21. James MK, Vuong A, Grizzle MK, Schuster SV, Shaffer JE (1992) Hemodynamic effects of GI 87084B, an ultra-short acting mu-opioid analgesic, in anesthetized dogs. J Pharmacol Exp Ther 263:84-91
22. DeSouza G, Lewis MC, TerRiet MF (1997) Severe bradycardia after remifentanil [letter]. Anesthesiology 87:1019-20
23. Reitan JA, Stengert KB, Wymore ML, Martucci RW (1978) Central vagal control of fentanyl-induced bradycardia during halothane anesthesia. Anesth Analg 57:31-6

24. Sebel PS, Hoke JF, Westmoreland C, Hug CC, Jr., Muir KT, Szlam F (1995) Histamine concentrations and hemodynamic responses after remifentanil. Anesth Analg 80:990-3
25. Ogilvy AJ (1998) Awareness during total intravenous anaesthesia with propofol and remifentanil [letter]. Anaesthesia 53:308
26. Egan TD, Lemmens HJ, Fiset P, Hermann DJ, Muir KT, Stanski DR, Shafer SL (1993) The pharmacokinetics of the new short-acting opioid remifentanil (GI87084B) in healthy adult male volunteers [see comments]. Anesthesiology 79:881-92
27. Westmoreland CL, Hoke JF, Sebel PS, Hug CC, Jr., Muir KT (1993) Pharmacokinetics of remifentanil (GI87084B) and its major metabolite (GI90291) in patients undergoing elective inpatient surgery [see comments]. Anesthesiology 79:893-903
28. Chism JP, Rickert DE (1996) The pharmacokinetics and extra-hepatic clearance of remifentanil, a short-acting opioid agonist, in male beagle dogs during constant rate infusions. Drug Metab Dispos 24:34-40
29. Duthie DJ, Stevens JJ, Doyle AR, Baddoo HH, Gupta SK, Muir KT, Kirkham AJ (1997) Remifentanil and pulmonary extraction during and after cardiac anesthesia. Anesth Analg 84:740-4
30. Hughes MA, Glass PS, Jacobs JR (1992) Context-sensitive half-time in multicompartment pharmacokinetic models for intravenous anesthetic drugs [see comments]. Anesthesiology 76:334-41
31. Shafer SL, Varvel JR (1991) Pharmacokinetics, pharmacodynamics, and rational opioid selection. Anesthesiology 74:53-63
32. Egan TD (1997) The clinical pharmacology of the new fentanyl congeners. International Anesthesia Research Society 1997 Review Course Lectures (Anesth Analg Supplement) 31-38
33. Minto CF, Schnider TW, Shafer SL (1997) Pharmacokinetics and pharmacodynamics of remifentanil. II. Model application. Anesthesiology 86:24-33
34. Davis PJ, Lerman J, Suresh S, McGowan FX, Cote CJ, Landsman I, Henson LG (1997) A randomized multicenter study of remifentanil compared with alfentanil, isoflurane, or propofol in anesthetized pediatric patients undergoing elective strabismus surgery. Anesth Analg 84:982-9
35. Davis PJ, Ross AK, Henson LG, Muir KT (1997) Remifentanil pharmacokinetics in neonates. Anesthesiology 87:A1064
36. Egan TD, Huizinga B, Gupta SK, Jaarsma RL, Sperry RJ, Yee JB, Muir KT (1998) Remifentanil pharmacokinetics in obese versus lean elective surgery patients. Anesthesiology (in press):
37. Roubenoff R, Kehayias JJ (1991) The meaning and measurement of lean body mass. Nutr Rev 49:163-75

38. Hoke JF, Shlugman D, Dershwitz M, Michalowski P, Malthouse Dufore S, Connors PM, Martel D, Rosow CE, Muir KT, Rubin N, Glass PS (1997) Pharmacokinetics and pharmacodynamics of remifentanil in persons with renal failure compared with healthy volunteers. Anesthesiology 87:533-41

39. Rosow C (1993) Remifentanil: a unique opioid analgesic [editorial; comment]. Anesthesiology 79:875-6

40. Dershwitz M, Hoke JF, Rosow CE, Michalowski P, Connors PM, Muir KT, Dienstag JL (1996) Pharmacokinetics and pharmacodynamics of remifentanil in volunteer subjects with severe liver disease. Anesthesiology 84:812-20

41. Navapurkar VU, S. A, Frazer NM, Gupta SK, Muir KT, Park GR (1995) Pharmacokinetics of remifentanil during hepatic transplantation. Anesthesiology 83:A382

42. Stiller RL, Davis PJ, McGowan FX (1995) In vitro metabolism of remifentanil: the effects of pseudocholinesterase deficiency. Anesthesiology 83:A381

43. Kharasch ED, Thummel KE (1993) Human alfentanil metabolism by cytochrome P450 3A3/4. An explanation for the interindividual variability in alfentanil clearance? Anesth Analg 76:1033-9

44. Kharasch ED, Russell M, Mautz D, Thummel KE, Kunze KL, Bowdle A, Cox K (1997) The role of cytochrome P450 3A4 in alfentanil clearance. Implications for interindividual variability in disposition and perioperative drug interactions. Anesthesiology 87:36-50

45. Wrighton SA, Ring BJ, Watkins PB, VandenBranden M (1989) Identification of a polymorphically expressed member of the human cytochrome P-450III family. Mol Pharmacol 36:97-105

46. Vuyk J, Mertens MJ, Olofsen E, Burm AG, Bovill JG (1997) Propofol anesthesia and rational opioid selection: determination of optimal EC50-EC95 propofol-opioid concentrations that assure adequate anesthesia and a rapid return of consciousness. Anesthesiology 87:1549-62

47. Schuttler J, Albrecht S, Breivik H, Osnes S, Prys Roberts C, Holder K, Chauvin M, Viby Mogensen J, Mogensen T, Gustafson I, Lof L, Noronha D, Kirkham AJ (1997) A comparison of remifentanil and alfentanil in patients undergoing major abdominal surgery [see comments]. Anaesthesia 52:307-17

48. Cartwright DP, Kvalsvik O, Cassuto J, Jansen JP, Wall C, Remy B, Knape JT, Noronha D, Upadhyaya BK (1997) A randomized, blind comparison of remifentanil and alfentanil during anesthesia for outpatient surgery. Anesth Analg 85:1014-9

49. Kovac AL, Azad SS, Steer P, Witkowski T, Batenhorst R, McNeal S (1997) Remifentanil versus alfentanil in a balanced anesthetic technique for total abdominal hysterectomy. J Clin Anesth 9:532-41

50. Stevens JB, Wheatley L (1998) Tracheal intubation in ambulatory surgery patients: using remifentanil and propofol without muscle relaxants. Anesth Analg 86:45-9

51. Munday IT, Ward PM, Sorooshian S, Stafford MA, Jones RM, Hull CJ, Shaikh S (1995) Interaction between remifentanil and isoflurane in spontaneously breathing patients during ambulatory surgery. Anesthesiology 83:A23

52. Jhaveri R, Joshi P, Batenhorst R, Baughman V, Glass PS (1997) Dose comparison of remifentanil and alfentanil for loss of consciousness. Anesthesiology 87:253-9

53. Lauwers MH, Vanlersberghe C, Camu F (1998) Comparison of remifentanil and propofol infusions for sedation during regional anesthesia. Reg Anesth Pain Med 23:64-70

54. Gold MI, Watkins WD, Sung YF, Yarmush J, Chung F, Uy NT, Maurer W, Clarke MY, Jamerson BD (1997) Remifentanil versus remifentanil/midazolam for ambulatory surgery during monitored anesthesia care. Anesthesiology 87:51-7

55. Avramov MN, Smith I, White PF (1996) Interactions between midazolam and remifentanil during monitored anesthesia care. Anesthesiology 85:1283-9

56. Hoffman WE, Cunningham F, James MK, Baughman VL, Albrecht RF (1993) Effects of remifentanil, a new short-acting opioid, on cerebral blood flow, brain electrical activity, and intracranial pressure in dogs anesthetized with isoflurane and nitrous oxide. Anesthesiology 79:107-13

57. Warner DS, Hindman BJ, Todd MM, Sawin PD, Kirchner J, Roland CL, Jamerson BD (1996) Intracranial pressure and hemodynamic effects of remifentanil versus alfentanil in patients undergoing supratentorial craniotomy. Anesth Analg 83:348-53

58. Guy J, Hindman BJ, Baker KZ, Borel CO, Maktabi M, Ostapkovich N, Kirchner J, Todd MM, Fogarty Mack P, Yancy V, Sokoll MD, McAllister A, Roland C, Young WL, Warner DS (1997) Comparison of remifentanil and fentanyl in patients undergoing craniotomy for supratentorial space-occupying lesions. Anesthesiology 86:514-24

59. Johnson KB, Egan TD (1998) Remifentanil and propofol combination for awake craniotomy: case report with pharmacokinetic simulations. J Neurosurg Anesthesiol 10:25-9

60. Russell D, Royston D, Rees PH, Gupta SK, Kenny GN (1997) Effect of temperature and cardiopulmonary bypass on the pharmacokinetics of remifentanil. Br J Anaesth 79:456-9

61. Michelsen LG, Hug CC, Woda RP, Howie MB, Porembka DT, Kirkhart BA (1996) Early extubation of CABG patients after remifentanil anesthesia. Anesth Analg 82:S314

62. Lynn AM (1996) Remifentanil: the pediatric anaesthetist's opiate? Paediatr Anaesth 6:433-435

63.   Kan RE, Hughes SC, Rosen MA, Kessin C, Preston PG, Lobo EP (1998) Intravenous remifentanil: placental transfer, maternal and neonatal effects. Anesthesiology 88:1467-1474

64.   Brada SA, Egan TD, Viscomi CM (1998) The use of remifentanil infusion to facilitate epidural catheter placement in a parturient: a case report with pharmacokinetic simulations. Int J Obstet Anesth 7:124-127

65.   Bowdle TA, Ready LB, Kharasch ED, Nichols WW, Cox K (1997) Transition to post-operative epidural or patient-controlled intravenous analgesia following total intravenous anaesthesia with remifentanil and propofol for abdominal surgery. Eur J Anaesthesiol 14:374-9

66.   Bowdle TA, Camporesi EM, Maysick L, Hogue CW, Jr., Miguel RV, Pitts M, Streisand JB (1996) A multicenter evaluation of remifentanil for early postoperative analgesia. Anesth Analg 83:1292-7

DRUG ADDICTION AMONG ANESTHESIOLOGISTS

Mervyn Maze

Incidence of Addiction among Stanford Anesthesia Residents

1980 - 1995
Graduates   220

Addicted   19

Outcome of Addicted Residents

Good   14

Poor   5

Dead   3

Death due to other causes   1

Incidence of Addiction in the Specialty

- **Ongoing ASA Prospective Study**
  - 135 confirmed cases/19.547 person years
  - 28% were AOA
  - 32% have family history
  - 12% joined residency with a prior history
  - 88% are male
- **Physicians undergoing treatment in Georgia**
  - 33.7% are Anesthesia Residents

T. H. Stanley and T. D. Egan (eds.), Anesthesia for the New Millennium, 263–266.

Definitions - Disease Model

- **Addiction**
    - chronic compulsive use despite destructive consequences
- **Dependence**
    - Physical:
    * tolerance
    * withdrawal
    - Psychologic
    * craving for positive effects
    * avoiding negative effects
- **Substance Abuse**
    - use of psychoactive substance
    - detrimental to individual or society

Etiology

- **predisposing personality**
- **drug availability**
- **circumstances bringing these together**
- job stress
- "Rodney Dangerfield" syndrome
- therapeutic optimism

Clinical Manifestations

- Unusual changes or frequently swings in behavior
- Withdrawal from family, friends, !eisure activities
- When confronted, vehemently rejects activities
- Domestic disharmony
- Need to be near their drug source
  - alcoholics absent from work
  - opiate narcotics users spend additional hrs in hospital
- Usually maintain well at work (- anesthetic record)
- Always wear gowns
- Frequent health complaints

Evaluation of Potential Impairment

- Investigate-verification
  - drug use
  - drug diversion
  - behavioral aberrations
- Intervention
  - team of non-judgmental, supportive peers
  - highly structured and stylized
- Referral for diagnosis and treatment

Re-entry into Anesthesiology

- **Consider a different specialty if narcotic abuser**
  - 49% relapse rate
  - 17% mortality rate
  - 34% success
- **Re-entry contract**
  - abstention
  - monitoring
- **Attendance at self-help groups**

Prevention

- **Drug control**
- **Education**
- **Pre-employment and random drug screens**
- **Stress management**

ANTAGONISM OF ANESTHETIC EFFECTS

Pierre Fiset

The nature of anesthetic practice is such that a rapid and complete reversal of drug effect is often needed. The introduction of new pharmacological agents with favorable and rapid recovery curves is welcome because it allows us to change the level of effect very quickly and insures a faster disappearance of effect and fewer unwanted residual effects like partial paralysis, undue sedation or respiratory depression. Nevertheless, because longer acting agents are still used in many cases, antagonistic compounds are still needed. The present review will cover the antagonism of muscle relaxants, benzodiazepines, narcotics, and a very peculiar form of antagonism of anesthetic effects seen after the administration of physostigmine (Antilirium®).

MUSCLE RELAXANTS

Muscle relaxants exert their action by competing with acetylcholine (ACh) at the muscarinic receptor of the neuromuscular junction. They are of two types: non-depolarizing and depolarizing.

Non-depolarizing muscle relaxants bind to the nicotinic receptor at the neuro-muscular junction and prevent the opening of the ion channel responsible for the initiation and propagation of the muscle fiber contraction, resulting in muscle paralysis. They also bind non-specifically to the muscarinic and nicotinic ACh receptors of autonomic ganglionic cells and the sinus node of the heart. The relative affinity of this extra-muscular binding will determine the magnitude of side effects (cardiac dysrhythmia or hypotension) of a specific muscle relaxant. Histamine release is another factor that significantly contributes to hypotension.

T. H. Stanley and T. D. Egan (eds.), Anesthesia for the New Millennium, 267–275.

Muscle relaxants can be conveniently classified according to their duration of action:

Short	Intermediate	Long Acting
Mivacurium	Vecuronium	Pancuronium
	Atracurium	d-Tubocurarine
	Rocuronium	Doxacurium
	Cisatracurium	Pipecuronium

Since the binding of the muscle relaxant is competitive, the strategy for reversal of effect is to increase the availability of ACh at the level of the receptor. This is accomplished by the administration of anticholinesterase drugs that will inhibit acetylcholinesterase (AChE), the enzyme responsible for the breakdown of ACh, and thereby increase the lifetime of ACh in the synaptic cleft and the probability that it will displace the muscle relaxant from the binding site. AChE inhibitors also have pre-junctional and direct muscarinic effects that can modulate the classical mode of action. Like that of muscle relaxants, their action is not restricted to the nicotinic receptor of the muscle membrane. To avoid important muscarinic side effects (mainly bradycardia), AChE inhibitors are always co-administered with an antimuscarinic: atropine or glycopyrrolate.

Three AChE inhibitors are currently used for muscle relaxant reversal: neostigmine, edrophonium and pyridostigmine. The speed and completeness of reversal are influenced by several factors (1,2).

Depth of Blockade

The magnitude of neuromuscular blockade is conveniently assessed by the administration of train-of-four electrical stimulation of a peripheral nerve and monitoring of the evoked muscular response. Ideally, we aim at maintaining one twitch response, which corresponds to a 90 to 95% degree of blockade. When a deeper blockade is achieved, corresponding to an absence of twitch response, post-tetanic count stimulation is used to evaluate recovery times.

When a standard dose of reversal is used, a deep block will take longer to reverse. In fact, the maximum effect of neostigmine is reached within 10 minutes (3). If maximum reversal is not obtained at that time, further reversal is dependent on the clearance of the muscle relaxant from the effect site. This process is slower with longer acting muscle relaxants. For a very deep block, neostigmine seems to be preferable to edrophonium (4,5).

Antagonist Administered

The speed of onset for a moderate depth (1 twitch) of blockage is: edrophonium > neostigmine > pyridostigmine.

Dose of Antagonist

Increasing the dose of AChE inhibitors will increase the speed and efficiency of recovery only to a certain point. When doses of 60 to 80 mgΣkg^{-1} of neostigmine and 1.0 to 1.5 mgΣkg^{-1} have been given, the maximal effect occurs within 10 minutes and further recovery depends mainly on the rate of clearance of the relaxant. Higher doses are not recommended.

Concentration of Inhaled Anesthetic

Since the effect of muscle relaxants is enhanced by inhalation anesthetics, is makes sense to expect that reversal will also be delayed if the residual concentration of inhaled agents is high. A few studies have been published to support this fact (6,7).

Special Circumstances

Acid-base balance, electrolyte imbalance (Ca++), and underlying diseases like myasthenia gravis or myotonia are all factors that can influence the reversal of muscle relaxants.

Clinical Implications

The decision to reverse a muscle relaxant is most of the time based on the evaluation of the train-of-four ratio (T4/T1 response) while the patient is still under anesthesia. A TOF ratio of 0.7 has been correlated with an absence of clinical weakness or respiratory impairment (8,9). Unfortunately, a number of studies have shown that visual or even tactile (10,11) evaluation of the TOF ratio is often misleading such that residual curarization could be easily missed. I usually reverse any patient having received long-acting muscle relaxants. When I use intermediate-acting muscle relaxants, if I evaluate that the TOF ratio is > 0.7 (I may be wrong!!!!), I do not give reversal, but I carefully evaluate the patient in the O.R. after extubation to ascertain that he/she meets all clinical criteria of recovery. If I have doubts, I administer AChE inhibitors.

Finally, it is worth noting that after succinylcholine, a phase II block can be reversed by the administration of AChE inhibitors.

OPIOID ANTAGONISM

Opioid receptor pharmacology has grown very complex, and it is beyond the scope of this review to cover the whole subject. Instead, we will focus on the use of naloxone and nalbuphine in the context of anesthesia and post-operative pain management.

Most opioids used in anesthesia (e.g., morphine, fentanyl, alfentanil, sufentanil and remifentanil) exert their action by binding with the m receptor, which causes analgesia, bradycardia, sedation, respiratory depression, euphoria and physical dependence. Despite an increased margin of safety during balanced anesthesia due to controlled ventilation, the level of narcotization has to be carefully titrated so that at the end of surgery the patient is awake, spontaneously breathing, and has reasonable pain control. After emergence the margin of safety for adequate pain control and sufficient respiratory drive is small and depends on factors like the importance of surgical pain, time from surgery, and other individual factors like age, tolerance, or physiological condition. Opioid antagonists may be used to reverse respiratory depression in the context of recovery following anesthesia, or following the administration of neuraxial opioids or PCA for post-operative pain.

The most widely used opioid antagonist is naloxone. It is an antagonist to the mu, delta, kappa, and sigma receptors. It is a competitive antagonist, so that when a certain proportion of receptors is occupied by an agonist, careful titration will result in the desired level of reversal. It is thus possible to reverse opioid-induced respiratory depression without completely reversing the analgesic effects. Naloxone's pharmacokinetic/dynamic profile results in a fairly rapid onset, but also a rapid disappearance from the receptor, such that its duration of effect will not match that of long-acting agonists like morphine and sufentanil. Renarcotization may occur, resulting in a reinstallation of respiratory depression.

Although careful titration may result in a favorable clinical outcome, naloxone can cause hypertension, tachycardia and other significant hemodynamic alterations that may be explained by a sudden onset of pain, rapid awakening, and even non-specific sympathetic activation. This should be remembered if one considers the use of naloxone in patients with coronary artery disease, hypertension or cerebrovascular diseases. Case reports of pulmonary edema, severe hypertensive episodes, cardiac dysrhythmia and arrest have also been reported, even after small doses (12) (80 mg) and in an unpredictable context.

It follows that even if naloxone may indeed be a very useful, lifesaving drug, it should be used scarcely and with great caution. Bailey and Stanley, in Miller's Anesthesia, 4th Edition, propose the following rules:

1) Use opioids in anesthesia in such a way that reversal agents are rarely necessary.
2) Avoid inducing unnecessary intraoperative hypocapnia, so that body carbon dioxide stores will not be depleted and adequate ventilatory drive will remain after anesthesia and surgery.
3) Carefully titrate opioid antagonists.
4) Avoid reversal agents in patients with hypertension or with cardiac or cerebrovascular disease.

When needed, the 0.4 mg ampule of naloxone may be diluted in 10 cc of saline and administered by 0.5 to 1 cc increments every 2 to 3 minutes. In my institution, a naloxone ampule is attached to every PCA or epidural pump. Naloxone is also a standing order for respiratory depression following bolus administration of epidural morphine.

Nalbuphine could be an alternative to naloxone in certain circumstances. It has antagonistic properties at the mu receptor and is an agonist of the kappa receptor. This complex pattern of action may result in a significant analgesia (10 mg nalbuphine = 10 mg morphine) coupled with a ceiling effect on respiratory depression. Unfortunately, higher doses do not seem to result in improved analgesia, so that a ceiling effect of analgesic action also seems to exist. Bailey (13) failed to reverse morphine-induced respiratory depression with nalbuphine.

BENZODIAZEPINE ANTAGONISM

Benzodiazepines (BZD) act by binding with the BZD receptor that is located on the g_2-subunit of the g-aminobutyric acid (GABA)$_A$ receptor. This results in a modulatory enhancement of the effect of GABA, the major inhibitory neurotransmitter in the brain, to cause anxiolytic, anticonvulsant and muscle relaxation effects. High doses, as the ones used for induction of anesthesia, will cause hypnosis.

The effects of BZD can be reversed rapidly and completely by the competitive antagonist flumazenil. Flumazenil has very little, if any, effect of its own on CNS function. It has no known toxic potential, and its action is specific to the BZD receptor. Reversal is dose dependent and is very rapid (15).

Flumazenil does not antagonize other anesthetic agents like barbiturates, opioids, ketamine, or inhalational agents. It has been used anecdotally with some success to alleviate symptoms related to hepatic encephalopathy.

Although Flumazenil can completely reverse BZD effects, its pharmacokinetic/pharmacodynamic characteristics will result in an early termination of action compared to midazolam, diazepam or lorazepam. Resedation can occur after a bolus, necessitating repeat doses or the use of an infusion that will be titrated according to the clinical picture.

The initial bolus should be between 0.2 to 0.5 mg, and repeat doses may be administered if needed. If no effect is seen after 2 mg, the clinician should be looking for causes other than BZD to explain excessive sedation. Flumazenil should be used with caution, if at all in, epileptic patients and in individuals using BZD chronically.

REVERSAL OF SEDATION BY PHYSOSTIGMINE

Drugs which specifically effect cholinergic transmission, and which also have an effect on the level of consciousness, have a long history of use by anesthesiologists. Physostigmine was shown to decrease the time required for return to consciousness following anaesthesia with halothane (16) and ketamine (17). Physostigmine was also shown to rapidly reverse prolonged postoperative somnolence following induction of anaesthesia with midazolam (18) and was reported to diminish the time to recover

273

cognitive function following sedation induced by meperidine, propiomazine and scopolamine administered to parturients (19). A case report describes a patient who demonstrated delayed arousal following administration of halothane and in whom physostigmine produced abrupt awakening after two minutes (20). Interestingly, physostigmine has also been reported to antagonize the respiratory depressant effect of morphine (21). Physostigmine has recently been shown to increase the dose of propofol required to induce loss of consciousness (22).

Our research group has started to investigate more rigorously the modulatory effect of cholinergic drugs on anesthetics. In a group of volunteers, we have induced and maintained unconsciousness with an infusion of propofol and have attempted reversal with physostigmine. Unconsciousness was reversed clinically and objectively (BIS and ASSR) in 9/10 subjects (23). In another group of subjects, the reversal was blocked by pre-administration of scopolamine, an anticholinergic drug that crossed the blood-brain barrier (24). We are currently repeating the experiments with other classes of anesthetic drugs and are using Positron Emission Tomography to determine muscarinic receptor occupancy.

Clearly, physostigmine's effect is not explained by agonist/antagonist competitive mechanisms. Central cholinergic transmission is affected directly or indirectly by anesthetic drugs and may play a central role in the generation of anesthetic action.

BIBLIOGRAPHY

1. Savarese JJ, Miller RD, Lien CA, Caldwell JE: Pharmacology of muscle relaxants and their antagonists. Anesthesia. Edited by Miller RD. New York, Churchill Livingstone, 1994, pp 417-87
2. Bevan DR, Donati F, Kopman AF: Reversal of neuromuscular blockade. Anesthesiology 77:785-805, 1992
3. Beemer GH, Bjorksten AR, Dawson PJ: Determinants of the reversal time of competitive neuromuscular blockade by anticholinesterase drugs. Br J Anesth 66:469, 1991
4. Donati F, Lahoud J, McCready D, Bevan DR: Neostigmine, pyridostigmine and edrophonium as antagonists of moderate and profound atracurium blockade. Can J Anaesth 34:589-93, 1987
5. Rupp SM, McChristen J, Miller RD: Neostigmine and edrophonium antagonism of varying intensity of neuromuscular blockade by atracurium, pancuronium or vecuronium. Anesthesiology 64:711, 1986

6.   Delisle S, Bevan DR: Impaired neostigmine antagonism of pancuronium during enflurane anesthesia in man. Br J Anaesth 54:441, 1982

7.   Baurain MJ, D'Hollander AA, Melot C: Effects of residual concentrations of isoflurane on the reversal of vecuronium-induced neuromuscular blockade. Anesthesiology 74:474, 1991

8.   Ali HH, Wilson RS, Savarese JJ, Kitz RJ: The effect of tubocurarine on indirectly elicited train-of-four muscle response and respiratory measurements in humans. Br J Anaesth 47:570-4, 1975

9.   Brand JB, Cullen DJ, Wilson NE, Ali HH: Spontaneous recovery from nondepolarizing neuromuscular blockade: Correlation between clinical and evoked responses. Anesth Analg 56:55-8, 1977

10. Thomas PD, Worthlet LIG, Russell WJ: How useful is visual and tactile assessment of neuromuscular blockade using a peripheral nerve stimulator? Anaesth Intensive Care 12:6869, 1984

11. Dupuis JY, Martin R, Tessonnier JM, Tetrault JP: Clinical assessment of the muscular response to tetanic nerve stimulation. Can J Anaesth 37:397-400, 1990

12. Partridge BL, Ward CF: Pulmonary edema following low-dose naloxone administration. Anesthesiology 65:709-10, 1986

13. Bailey PL, Clark NJ, Pace NL, et al: Failure of nalbuphine to antagonize morphine. Anesth Analg 65:605, 1986

14. Mendelson WB: Neuropharmacology of sleep induction by benzodiazepines. Neurobiology 16:221, 1992

15. Fiset P, Lemmens HLM, Egan TE, Shafer SL, Stanski DR: Pharmacodynamic modeling of the electroencephalographic effects of flumazenil in healthy volunteers sedated with midazolam.   Clin Pharmacol Ther 58:567-82, 1995

16. Hill GE, Stanley TH, Sentker CR: Physostigmine reversal of postoperative somnolence. Can J Anaesth 24:707-11, 1977

17. Toro-Matos A, Rendon-Platas AM, Avila-Valdez E, Villarreal-Guzman RA: Physostigmine antagonizes ketamine. Anesth Analg 59:764-7, 1980

18. Caldwell CB, Gross JB: Physostigmine reversal of midazolam-induced sedation. Anesthesiology 57:125-7, 1982

19. Smith DB, Clark RB, Stephens SR, Sherman RL, Hyde ML: Physostigmine reversal of sedation in parturients.   Anesth Analg 55:478-80, 1976

20. Artru AA, Hui GS: Physostigmine reversal of general anesthesia for intraoperative neurological testing: associated EEG changes. Anesth Analg 65:1059-62, 1986

21. Snir-Mor I, Weinstock M, Davidson JT, Bahar M: Physostigmine antagonizes morphine-induced respiratory depression in human subjects. Anesthesiology 59:6-9, 1983

22. Fassoulaki A, Sarantopoulos C, Derveniotis C: Physostigmine increases the dose of propofol required to induce anaesthesia. Can J Anaesth 44:1148-51, 1997

23. Meuret P, Backman S, Bonhomme V, Plourde G, Fiset P: Effect of physostigmine on propofol-induced loss of consciousness and changes in evoked auditory responses in man. Society for Neuroscience 1997(Abstract)

24. Bonhomme V, Meuret P, Backman SB, Plourde G, Fiset P: Cholinergic mechanisms mediating propofol-induced loss of consciousness. Can J Anaesth 45:A52-B1998 (Abstract)

ECONOMICS OF ANESTHESIA EDUCATION

Peter S. Sebel

INTRODUCTION

The costs of education are increasing. Since 1960, medical student tuition has grown by 400% for private schools and 250% for public schools, adjusted for inflation (1). Once educated, there is a contention that physicians' income is unfairly distributed and that there are disparities between generalists and specialists (2-5). It has also been suggested that physicians' income is too high in general (6).

There is obviously no absolute standard to judge the appropriateness of physicians' income in the United States. Various techniques have been suggested: historical comparisons, comparisons with physicians' incomes in other countries, or comparisons of incomes of other professionals (7).

The Association of American Medical Colleges has examined the indebtedness of United States medical students (8). They found that over the past decade, that in constant dollars, the average indebtedness of students graduating from public schools increased by 59.2% and from private school 64.2%. Debts in excess of $100,000.00 at graduation are not uncommon. Entering medical students have declared their intention to rely more heavily on loans as a means of financing. These findings suggest that students may be throwing caution to the wind in the more favorable climate for borrowing and ignoring indicators of changing practice opportunities and reduced incomes ahead.

Weeks and colleagues (9) carried out a comparison on the return of educational investment for people in business, law, dentistry, and medicine (both primary care and procedure-based specialties). They used standard financial analysis techniques to examine the calculated return on

T. H. Stanley and T. D. Egan (eds.), Anesthesia for the New Millennium, 277–283.

education investment for high school graduates who chose amongst the five careers. They adjusted for the difference in average number of hours worked in each profession and calculated a net present value of the educational investment, adjusted for the average difference in hours worked. They found that the annual yield on the educational investment over a working life was 15.9% for primary care physicians, 29% for business people, 25.4% for attorneys, 20.9% for specialist physicians, and 20.7% for dentists. As anesthesiologists and nurse anesthetists debate the relative supervisory and billing status of their respective professions, this analysis was undertaken to determine the relative returns on the educational investment for the two career choices.

We also sought to determine how many years after obtaining a Bachelor's degree does the cumulative income of an anesthesiologist exceed that of an anesthetist.

METHODS

The costs of education were obtained by surveying 12 anesthesiologists and 18 anesthetists in order to determine:

> Date of Bachelor's degree
> Date of postgraduate degree
> Private/public institutions
> Tuition and living expenses per year
> Educational debt information

These data were used to determine the tuition fees and cost of living during the educational period for each returned survey. Since each year of graduation was different, the dollar cost of education was calculated in 1996 equivalent dollar levels as follows:

Educational costs of private and public institutions were obtained from the National Center for Educational Statistics for the years 1965-1996. Costs of education were plotted against year of education and regression analysis performed to determine the relationship between cost and year (see Results). The following equation was then used to convert the educational cost to 1996 dollars:

$$\text{Cost in 19xx} = \frac{\text{NCES \$ for 1996 (Public / Private)}}{\text{Solution to quadratic function for 19xx}}$$

In order to reflect comparable education costs, all tuition and living expenses were assumed to have been borrowed at 8% interest. Loans were assumed to accumulate to graduation (anesthetists) or completion of residency (anesthesiologists). These loans were then assumed to have been paid back over 10 years at 8% interest.

In order to estimate income for anesthetists, the Emory salary scale was used. This was incremented from the bottom of the scale to the top of the scale over 10 years with an extra 20% to allow for shift differentials/overtime. For physicians' salaries, data from the Graduate Medical Education Office was used to calculate residents' salaries, and for anesthesiologists' salaries, data from the American Association of Medical Colleges (Southern Region) were used. Physicians were assumed to undertake a four-year residency and then to progress from the 20th percentile of assistant professor to the 50th percentile of associate professor over 10 years. For anesthesiologists and anesthetists, the cumulative income minus loan repayments over a 20-year period was calculated. Year 1 was considered the first year after completing the Bachelor's degree.

RESULTS

Educational costs in the years 1965-1996 for both private and public institutions were found to fit a quadratic function (r^2=0.998 in both cases). See Figures 1 and 2.

The educational cost data from our study varied significantly from the NCES costs (Table 1).

TABLE 1. OUR DATA vs. NATIONAL DATA FOR EDUCATIONAL INSTITUTIONS

OUR DATA: Calculated 1996 Costs Mean / SD	NATIONAL DATA: NCES Costs
Private $129,529/$70,946	$89,880
Public $80,431/38,873	$29,804

The total accumulated debt at time of completion of training related to type of institution is shown in Table 2.

TABLE 2. TOTAL ACCUMULATED DEBT

	Public	Private
Anesthetist	$152,164	$139,520
Anesthesiologist	$319,037	$572,035

The graph shows the total cumulative income (minus loan repayments) of anesthesiologists and anesthetists over 20 years. It is noteworthy that the cumulative income of anesthesiologists educated in public institutions exceeds that of anesthetists at 13 years, whereas those educated in private institutions exceeds that of anesthetists in 19 years. Table 3 shows the total return over 20 years and the annual return on investment (ROI).

TABLE 3. ANNUAL RETURN ON INVESTMENT (ROI)

	Total Investment	Total $ Return at 20 years	Annual Return on Investment
Anesthetist	$197,763	$1,228,980	31%
Anesthesiologist	$445,536	$1,625,375	18%

DISCUSSION

The data in this study tends to underestimate the difference in cumulative income between anesthesiologists and anesthetists. It fails to take into account the time value of money and the opportunity costs of the additional investment in physician training. Thus, it is clear that, in terms of the percentage return on investment, education as an anesthetist has a much better return than that of anesthesiologist.

Assuming all educational costs are borrowed, it takes an anesthesiologist who went to private schools 19 years until the estimated cumulative income exceeds that of an anesthetist.

Viewed strictly from the point of view of return on investment, it is clear that the nurse anesthetist has made the rational decision, in that the return on the investment is much higher. However, it can be argued that the physician anesthesiologist is relatively underpaid in his/her profession. The return on investment over twenty years does not match that of the nurse anesthetist and suggests that physician compensation should be increased in order to provide a reasonable rate of return on the costs of education.

Figure 1.

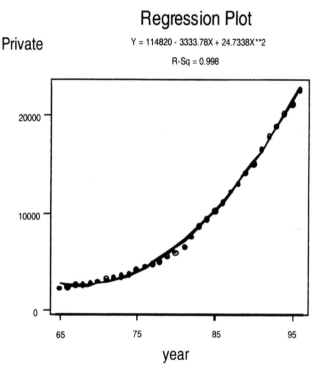

Regression Plot

Private

$Y = 114820 - 3333.78X + 24.7338X^{**}2$

R-Sq = 0.998

year

282

Figure 2.

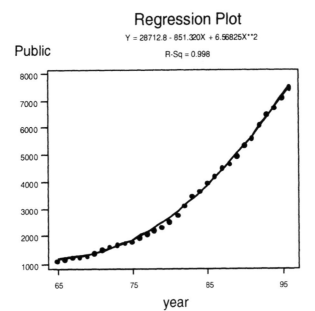

Regression Plot

Y = 28712.8 - 851.320X + 6.56825X**2

R-Sq = 0.998

Public

year

Figure 3.

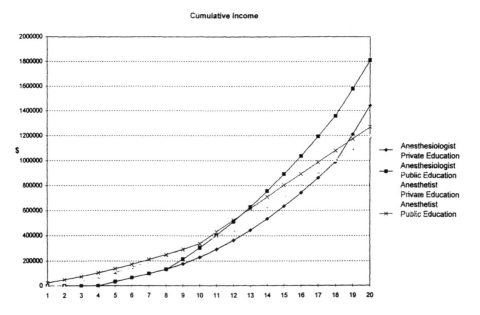

Cumulative Income

$

Anesthesiologist
Private Education

Anesthesiologist
Public Education

Anesthetist
Private Education

Anesthetist
Public Education

Year Since Bachelor's Degree

REFERENCES

1. Chhabra, A: Medical School Tuition and the Cost of Medical Education. JAMA 1996; 257(17):1372-1373
2. Schroder, SA, Sandy, LG: Specialty distribution of US physicians — the invisible driver of health care costs. N Engl J Med 1993; 328:961-3
3. Hsiao, WC, Braun, P, Becker E, et al: A national study of resource-based relative value scales for physician services: final report. Boston: Harvard School of Public Health, 1988
4. Hsiao, WC, Braun, P, Becker E, et al: Results and impacts of the Resource-Based Relative Value Scale. Med Care 1992;30:Suppl: NS61-NS79
5. Levy, JM, Borowitz, M, McNeill, S, London, WJ, Savord, G: Understanding the Medicare fee schedule and its impact on physicians under the final rule. Med Care 1992;30:Suppl:N280-NS94
6. Eckholm, E: Health plan is toughest on doctors making most. New York Times. November 7, 1993:26
7. Welch, HG, Fisher, ES: Let's make a deal: negotiating a settlement between physicians and society. N Engl J Med 1992;327:1312-5
8. Kassenbaum, DG, Szenas, PL, Schuchert, MK: On rising medical student debt: in for a penny, in for a pound. Acad Med 1996; Oct.:71(10):1124-34
9. Weeks, WB, Wallace, AE, Wallace, MM, Welch, HG: A Comparison of the Educational Costs and Incomes of Physicians and Other Professionals. N Engl J Med 1994;330(18):1280-6

THE ROLE OF KETAMINE IN ANESTHETIC PRACTICE

Paul F. White

Ketamine is a phencyclidine derivative that was synthesized by Stephens in 1963 (1). The first pharmacologic studies in humans were performed by Corssen and Domino in 1965. To describe the unique anesthetic state produced by ketamine, these investigators introduced the term "dissociative anesthesia" (2), a unique state of unconsciousness in which the patient is in a cataleptic trance-like state (often with their eyes open), disconnected from the surrounding environment, and apparently profoundly analgesic. The mechanism of ketamine's actions on the central nervous system (CNS) appears to be mediated through interactions with NMDA and non-NMDA glutamate receptors, as well as the kappa opioid receptors. However, NMDA-receptor antagonism accounts for the majority of the anesthetic, analgesic, amnestic, psychomimetic and neuroprotective effects of ketamine (3,4).

Clinical Uses

Since its introduction into clinical practice in the early 1970's, the clinical usefulness of ketamine has been limited because of its cardiovascular-stimulating properties and high incidence of psychomimetic emergence reactions. However, supplementation with other sedative-hypnotic drugs (e.g., diazepam, midazolam, thiopental, and propofol) has reduced the incidence of these untoward side effects. Therefore, ketamine has become a valuable drug in specific clinical situations (Table) (5). In addition to its clinical uses in the operating room, intensive care units, and emergency department, ketamine has proved valuable for diagnostic and therapeutic procedures in a wide variety of remote locations. Ketamine is an ideal anesthetic agent for anesthesia for catastrophic surgery (e.g., war, mass casualties, accidents, massive hemorrhage, inaccessibility to the victim's body). In the latter situations,

285

T. H. Stanley and T. D. Egan (eds.), Anesthesia for the New Millennium, 285–288.

ketamine can be given safely by a jet injector because of its high therapeutic index. In children, ketamine is well suited for magnetic resonance imaging because an infusion of ketamine can be easily titrated from a remote area. Given its pulmonary and circulatory effects, ketamine may be the anesthetic of choice in areas where trained anesthesiologists are not readily available during the performance of brief, painful

---

CLINICAL USES OF KETAMINE IN THE PRACTICE OF ANESTHESIOLOGY

Induction of anesthesia in high-risk patients:
    Shock or cardiovascular instability
    Severe dehydration
    Bronchospasm
    Severe anemia
    One-lung anesthesia
Obstetric patients:
    Induction of general anesthesia
        severe hypovolemia
        acute hemorrhage
        acute bronchospasm
    Low-dose for analgesia
        for "preemptive" analgesia
        to supplement regional anesthetic techniques
        at the time of delivery or during the postpartum period
Adjunct to local and regional anesthetic techniques:
    For sedation and analgesia during painful block procedures
    To supplement an inadequate block
Outpatient surgery:
    For brief diagnostic and therapeutic procedures
    To supplement local and regional block techniques
Use outside the operating room:
    In burn units (e.g., debridement, dressing changes)
    In emergency rooms (e.g., closed reductions)
    In intensive care units (e.g., sedation, painful procedures)
    In recovery rooms (e.g., postoperative sedation and analgesia)

procedures (e.g., for burn dressing changes, bone marrow biopsies and spinal taps in children, for insertion of invasive monitors, intubation for status asthmaticus, pericardiotomy). Recent studies would suggest that ketamine may possess unique preemptive analgesic effects as a result of its NMDA receptor blocking activity (6).

SUMMARY

Ketamine is a safe, rapid-acting, intravenous anesthetic and analgesic agent. Ketamine alone increases blood pressure and heart rate and produces profuse salivation, lacrimation, sweating, skeletal muscle hypertonus, involuntary purposeless movements, and agitation or even transient delirium during emergence (5). The use of a continuous infusion technique allows the anesthesiologist to titrate the drug more closely and thereby to reduce the total amount of drug required. Benzodiazepines are highly effective in preventing the marked cardiovascular responses and unpleasant emergence reactions associated with ketamine anesthesia. A combination of ketamine and midazolam was useful for rapid induction of anesthesia and can also be used for maintenance of anesthesia and sedation during total intravenous anesthesia (TIVA).

Numerous clinical studies have appeared in the literature over the last 15 years using ketamine infusion techniques. The clinical pharmacology and therapeutic uses of ketamine were initially reviewed in 1982 (7) and were subsequently updated in 1989 (8) and 1994 (5). Clinical applications for ketamine in anesthesia include a role in TIVA for major surgery, in the management of acute trauma, and in ambulatory surgery. Ketamine is widely used for sedation and analgesia during procedures using local anesthesia. In addition, ketamine can be used in intensive care units and emergency rooms for providing acute pain relief during brief procedures or painful manipulations. Although ketamine apparently does not possess all the physicochemical and pharmacologic properties of an ideal intravenous anesthetic (7), its diverse pharmacologic properties provide important insights in the continuing search for an intravenous drug that will be closer to the ideal. The availability of S(+) ketamine for clinical use would be a step in the right direction (9). However, this isomer of ketamine still possesses many of the side effects associated with the currently available racemic mixture. Future research should focus on the use of this unique anesthetic/analgesic compound as part of a "balanced" anesthetic technique to minimize its untoward side effects (10).

GENERAL REFERENCES

1. Corssen G: Historical aspects of ketamine: first clinical experience. In: Domino EF, ed. Status of ketamine in anesthesiology. NPP Books, 1990:1-5

2. Corssen G, Domino EF: Dissociative anesthesia: further pharmacologic studies and first clinical experience with the phencyclidine derivative CI-581. Anesth Analg 1966;42:29-40

3. Yamamura T, Harada K, Okamura A, Kemmotsu O: Is the site of action of ketamine anesthesia the N-methyl-D-aspartate receptor? Anesthesiology 1990;72:704-10

4. Irifune M, Shimizu T, Nomoto M, Fukuda T: Ketamine-induced anesthesia involves the N-methyl-D-aspartate receptor-channel complex in mice. Brain Res 1992;569:1-9

5. Gajraj N, White PF: Clinical pharmacology and applications of ketamine. In: Bowdle T, et al., eds. The pharmacologic basis of anesthesiology. New York: Churchill Livingstone, 1994:375-92

6. Fu ES, Miguel R, Scharf JE: Preemptive ketamine decreases postoperative narcotic requirements in patients undergoing abdominal surgery. Anesth Analg 1997;84:1086-90

7. White PF, Way WL, Trevor AJ: Ketamine: its pharmacology and therapeutic uses. Anesthesiology 1982;56:119-36

8. Reich DL, Silvay G. Ketamine: an update on the first twenty-five years of clinical experience. Can J Anaesth 1989;36:186

9. White PF, Ham J, Way WL, Trevor AJ: Pharmacology of ketamine isomers in surgical patients. Anesthesiology 1981;52:231-9

10. Bowdle A, Radant A, Cowley D, Kharasch E, et al: Psychedelic effects of ketamine in healthy volunteers. Anesthesiology 1998;88:82-8

DEVELOPMENTS IN
CRITICAL CARE MEDICINE AND ANESTHESIOLOGY

1. O. Prakash (ed.): *Applied Physiology in Clinical Respiratory Care.* 1982
    ISBN 90-247-2662-X
2. M.G. McGeown: *Clinical Management of Electrolyte Disorders.* 1983
    ISBN 0-89838-559-8
3. T.H. Stanley and W.C. Petty (eds.): *New Anesthetic Agents, Devices and Monitoring Techniques.* Annual Utah Postgraduate Course in Anesthesiology. 1983   ISBN 0-89838-566-0
4. P.A. Scheck, U.H. Sjöstrand and R.B. Smith (eds.): *Perspectives in High Frequency Ventilation.* 1983   ISBN 0-89838-571-7
5. O. Prakash (ed.): *Computing in Anesthesia and Intensive Care.* 1983   ISBN 0-89838-602-0
6. T.H. Stanley and W.C. Petty (eds.): *Anesthesia and the Cardiovascular System.* Annual Utah Postgraduate Course in Anesthesiology. 1984   ISBN 0-89838-626-8
7. J.W. van Kleef, A.G.L. Burm and J. Spierdijk (eds.): *Current Concepts in Regional Anaesthesia.* 1984   ISBN 0-89838-644-6
8. O. Prakash (ed.): *Critical Care of the Child.* 1984   ISBN 0-89838-661-6
9. T.H. Stanley and W.C. Petty (eds.): *Anesthesiology: Today and Tomorrow.* Annual Utah Postgraduate Course in Anesthesiology. 1985   ISBN 0-89838-705-1
10. H. Rahn and O. Prakash (eds.): *Acid-base Regulation and Body Temperature.* 1985
    ISBN 0-89838-708-6
11. T.H. Stanley and W.C. Petty (eds.): *Anesthesiology 1986.* Annual Utah Postgraduate Course in Anesthesiology. 1986   ISBN 0-89838-779-5
12. S. de Lange, P.J. Hennis and D. Kettler (eds.): *Cardiac Anaesthesia.* Problems and Innovations. 1986   ISBN 0-89838-794-9
13. N.P. de Bruijn and F.M. Clements: *Transesophageal Echocardiography.* With a contribution by R. Hill. 1987   ISBN 0-89838-821-X
14. G.B. Graybar and L.L. Bready (eds.): *Anesthesia for Renal Transplantation.* 1987
    ISBN 0-89838-837-6
15. T.H. Stanley and W.C. Petty (eds.): *Anesthesia, the Heart and the Vascular System.* Annual Utah Postgraduate Course in Anesthesiology. 1987   ISBN 0-89838-851-1
16. D. Reis Miranda, A. Williams and Ph. Loirat (eds.): *Management of Intensive Care.* Guidelines for Better Use of Resources. 1990   ISBN 0-7923-0754-2
17. T.H. Stanley (ed.): *What's New in Anesthesiology.* Annual Utah Postgraduate Course in Anesthesiology. 1988   ISBN 0-89838-367-6
18. G.M. Woerlee: *Common Perioperative Problems and the Anaesthetist.* 1988
    ISBN 0-89838-402-8
19. T.H. Stanley and R.J. Sperry (eds.): *Anesthesia and the Lung.* Annual Utah Postgraduate Course in Anesthesiology. 1989   ISBN 0-7923-0075-0
20. J. De Castro, J. Meynadier and M. Zenz: *Regional Opioid Analgesia.* Physiopharmacological Basis, Drugs, Equipment and Clinical Application. 1990   ISBN 0-7923-0162-5
21. J.F. Crul (ed.): *Legal Aspects of Anaesthesia.* 1989   ISBN 0-7923-0393-8

DEVELOPMENTS IN
CRITICAL CARE MEDICINE AND ANESTHESIOLOGY

22. E. Freye: *Cerebral Monitoring in the Operating Room and the Intensive Care Unit.* 1990
     ISBN 0-7923-0349-X

23. T.H. Stanley and R.J. Sperry (eds.): *Anesthesiology and the Heart.* Annual Utah Postgraduate
     Course in Anesthesiology. 1990   ISBN 0-7923-0634-1

24. T.H. Stanley, M.A. Ashburn, P. G. Fine (eds.): *Anesthesiology and Pain Management.* 1990
     ISBN 0-7923-1073-X

25. T.H. Stanley and R.J. Sperry (eds.): *Anesthesia and the Lung 1992.* Annual Utah Postgraduate
     Course in Anesthesiology. 1992   ISBN 0-7923-1563-4

26. G.M. Woerlee: *Kinetics and Dynamics of Intravenous Anesthetics.* 1992
     ISBN 0-7923-1506-5

27. A. Willner (ed.): *Cerebral Damage before and after Cardiac Surgery.* 1993
     ISBN 0-7923-1928-1

28. R.J. Sperry, J.O. Johnson and T.H. Stanley (eds.): *Anesthesia and the Central Nervous System.*
     Annual Utah Postgraduate Course in Anesthesiology. 1993   ISBN 0-7923-2083-2

29. T.H. Stanley and M.A. Ashburn (eds.): *Anesthesiology and Pain Management.* 1994
     ISBN 0-7923-2662-8

30. T.H. Stanley and P.G. Schafer (eds.): *Pediatric and Obstetrical Anesthesia.* Annual Utah
     Postgraduate Course in Anesthesiology. 1995   ISBN 0-7923-3346-2

31. T.H. Stanley and P.L. Bailey (eds.): *Anesthesiology and the Cardiovascular Patient.* 1996
     ISBN 0-7923-3895-2

32. J.O. Johnson, R.J. Sperry and T.H. Stanley (eds.): *Neuroanesthesia.* 1997
     ISBN 0-7923-4426-X

33. M.A. Ashburn, P.G. Fine and T.H. Stanley (eds.): *Pain Management and Anesthesiology.* 1998
     ISBN 0-7923-4995-4

34. T.H. Stanley and T.D. Egan (eds.): *Anesthesia for the New Millennium.* Modern Anesthetic
     Clinical Pharmacology. 1999   ISBN 0-7923-5632-2

KLUWER ACADEMIC PUBLISHERS – DORDRECHT / BOSTON / LONDON